# The Only Menopause Guide You'll Need

*A Johns Hopkins Press Health Book*

Second Edition

# The Only Menopause Guide You'll Need

*Michele Moore, M.D.*

THE JOHNS HOPKINS UNIVERSITY PRESS
*Baltimore and London*

*Note to the reader:* This book is not meant to substitute for medical care, and treatment should not be based solely on its contents. Treatment must be developed in a dialogue between the individual and her physician.

*Drug dosage:* The author and publisher have made reasonable efforts to determine that the selection and dosage of drugs discussed in this text conform to the practices of the general medical community. The medications described do not necessarily have specific approval by the U.S. Food and Drug Administration for use in the diseases and dosages for which they are recommended. In view of ongoing research, changes in governmental regulations, and the constant flow of information relating to drug therapy and drug reactions, the reader is urged to check the package insert of each drug for any change in indications and dosage and for warnings and precautions. This is particularly important when the recommended agent is a new and/or infrequently used drug.

© 2000, 2004 The Johns Hopkins University Press
All rights reserved. Published 2004
Printed in the United States of America on acid-free paper
9 8 7 6 5 4 3 2

The Johns Hopkins University Press
2715 North Charles Street
Baltimore, Maryland 21218-4363
www.press.jhu.edu

Library of Congress Cataloging-in-Publication Data
Moore, Michele.
The only menopause guide you'll need / Michele Moore.—2nd ed.
p. cm.
Includes bibliographical references and index.
ISBN 0-8018-8012-2 (alk. paper)—ISBN 0-8018-8013-0 (pbk. : alk. paper)
1. Menopause—Popular works. I. Title.
RG186.M66 2004
618.1'75—dc22          2004043483

A catalog record for this book is available from the British Library.

# Contents

# Preface

This book is the culmination of many hours spent with patients, hearing their stories, trying to alleviate their woes, and learning a great deal from them. Over the years I have come to believe that most women are heroines of a sort.

I also believe that this time in a woman's life is a natural phase of development, not a medical problem. I don't want to suggest that a woman's health care provider may not be sympathetic and helpful. Most health care providers, male and female, sincerely want to help with the "minor maladies" and risk factors associated with this phase of life. Needless to say, each woman will benefit from the guidance of her own trusted health care provider and the many published sources available to her. The final choice about taking action, however, is hers.

In this book I have tried to provide a framework of guidance and resources to help you make your difficult decisions. In my view, intervention—treatment—for the symptoms of menopause should not be offered routinely, but the availability of intervention should be made known to each woman and then initiated at her request. In Chapter 1, I touch on some of the symptoms of the three phases of menopause, while Chapter 2 takes up the health concerns that are particularly acute at this stage of life. Then, in Chapter 3, I begin the in-depth discussion of treatment options by providing an overview of the great variety of approaches to therapy, from allopathic and complementary to herbal and homeopathic medicine. Chapters 4, 5, and 6 explore the different approaches to therapy for the primary symptoms experienced by women in each of the three phases of menopause. Finally, in Chapters 7 and 8, I discuss the pros and cons of estriol and traditional hormone replacement therapy for women in perimenopause, menopause, and postmenopause.

Appendix 1 provides a quick guide to healthy diets, and Appendix 2 presents a patient's log, where you might want to record information about symptoms and any diagnostic tests or treatments you have tried. These are followed by a list of additional resources you may want to consult and a Glossary, with definitions of terms used in this book. At the end you'll find a list of references that I consulted in writing the book.

In my everyday work with women, it has become clear to me that I also wish to convey very specific advice. This is:

1. *Assess.* Remember that menopause is a normal, and inevitable, phase of life. Whether or not you actively do anything about it is best determined by an informed assessment of your own relative risks, on the one hand, and the advantages that may be offered by any action you take, on the other.

2. *Gather information.* Find out what you need to know in order to make an informed assessment of your potential risks and the potential advantages of action. Take what is right for you at this time and know that the rest exists.

3. *Make your own choice.* You have to live with it!

4. *Accept responsibility.* When you make the choice, you can take responsibility for it. We are women, not children.

5. *Reassess.* Every three to five years, reassess your situation. Life is not static. Your needs may change.

6. *Keep the spiritual and physical balance.* And remember, "this, too, shall pass."

One final note. In this book I have borrowed freely from my own experiences as well as those of my patients. To protect their privacy, I have altered names and details, but each woman will probably recognize herself. I hope that the very sincere fondness and respect that I have for them comes through.

# Acknowledgments

No book is ever written by a busy doctor without significant help from other people. In my case, I want to thank, first of all, my "office family." Gail Dubriske typed a first draft from my hen scratches on lots of sheets of paper. Both Esther Breckenridge, R.N., and Nyla Hiltz, R.N., read and critiqued the content as I produced it. Many thanks to Paul Dubriske, who gave generously of his time and encouragement.

At home, Chris, Martin, Anneke, and Mom were tolerant of the piles of reprints, journals, and manuscript pages littering our living room, as well as being generally supportive. My sister-in-law, Sue, boosted my ego by asking to read the first draft, and my friends MaryAnne Johnson and Judith Petry, M.D., both wrote me very encouraging notes after having read it.

Also, many thanks to Professor Moira O'Brien, who suggested I show the manuscript to academic publishers, and to Jacqueline Wehmueller, who championed it.

Last but far from least, thank you to all you special women who have shared your journeys with me over the years.

CHAPTER 1

# Symptoms You May Have Now
## Perimenopause, Menopause, and Postmenopause

I often joke with my patients about our return to adolescence, but there is more than a grain of truth in my joking. Surging hormones, whether they are due to puberty or to the menopausal stages, make us uncomfortable in both body and soul. We are moody and unpredictable and have close to zero tolerance for the foibles of others. We are also very uncertain about what is happening to us physiologically and whether or not the changes are normal. For many, the turmoil and bodily discomforts are compounded by a nagging sense that "maybe there's something wrong with me."

The good news is that the hormonal storms of both puberty and menopause are followed by times of greater calm and predictability. We can remember that we *did* survive puberty, and realize that we surely will also survive this developmental phase. Even those of us who experience our menopausal years while our daughters are adolescents will come through this! Accepting the inevitability of these phases is half the battle. Close communication with other women is the other half.

It has been pointed out that symptomatic menopause may be considered a cultural or psychological phenomenon. This is certainly interesting, and it may point to changes in our society that may eventually benefit women, but it is not helpful to the individual woman who is having difficulty here and now. To this woman, such observations may feel insulting and degrading. She lives in this culture and this way of life. The

1

woman who sails through this phase unscathed and unruffled is blessed and should be compassionate toward sisters less fortunate.

The cycles of a woman's life are not as clearly demarcated as the lists in Table 1 might make it seem. Rather, they are more like the phases of the moon, one shading *gradually* into the next. Technically, however, *menopause* (from the Greek word *mens,* meaning *monthly,* and *pausis,* meaning *cessation*) is defined as the cessation of menses. The term has expanded to include approximately one and a half to two years before and after cessation, however. The average age for menopause is still considered to be fifty-one, although we are seeing many women stop their periods much earlier. *Perimenopause* and *postmenopause* are terms used to describe the five to seven years before and the years after cessation of menses, but, again, these terms are used somewhat flexibly, as menopause is, really, a *process* that occurs over a number of years in a woman's life.

## Perimenopause

*Perimenopause* is a term that has been widely used only since about 1995. It refers to the time in a woman's life, usually five to seven years before she stops menstruating (but as early as ten years before), when the first symptoms of "wacky" hormones appear. The symptoms may include fatigue, memory problems, weight gain, short temper, bowel upset, sleep disruptions, and painful intercourse. Most women do not get all of these symptoms, and the severity of the symptoms can range from mild to severe.

For me the first symptom was fatigue, but, then, I could easily rationalize this: I had two small children, a busy office and hospital practice, and a Superwoman mentality that meant baking our bread, canning produce from our organic garden, being there for everyone. Before long, I felt totally inadequate and unable to perform to my own standards in any area of my life. I also felt as if this were a shameful secret I had to conceal. It was humiliating.

Gloria came in feeling every bit as humiliated and desperate as I remember feeling. Her problem was very personal, she said, and she told me: "I'm avoiding my husband. I stay up real late so he'll be asleep when I go up. I love him but I don't want sex. It's gotten so it hurts like a burning knife. He thinks I just don't want *him* any more, and we're starting to be distant with each other. I went to my regular doctor and he examined me and said everything was okay and maybe Hank and I should go to marriage counseling. I think I need a shrink but my girlfriend said to see you."

Sue has been sent to multiple specialists over the past two years. She was seeing a rheumatologist for her aching muscles and joints, and after all the test results proved to be normal, he told her that she probably had fibromyalgia, which would explain her difficulties with sleep, too. For her migraines, she was seeing a neurologist. The fatigue and depression were very understandable because of all the other problems. Why did it all come together in her forty-fifth year? Must be the stresses in her life. Finally, she began to have night sweats (and was tested for tuberculosis, because night sweats is one symptom of TB) and then hot flashes, and she skipped two periods. She now thought that she had a pretty good idea of what could be going on and asked her family doctor if she could be starting menopause. "No," he told her, "you're too young."

Because I hear so many stories like these, I now try to begin a dialogue about menopause with my patients when they are in their early forties. We usually just chat about the symptoms they may notice, and this becomes part of our "Bring me up to date" talk when they come in for a yearly exam. Sometimes my

Table 1. *Life Cycles of Adult Women*

| Puberty | Reproductive Years | Perimenopause | Menopause | Postmenopause |
|---|---|---|---|---|
| Menstrual irregularities: cramps, flooding | Menses more regular | Menstrual irregularities: erratic, spotting, cramps, flooding | Hot flashes | Hot flashes diminished |
| Sore breasts | Premenstrual stress | Weight gain | Night sweats | Night sweats diminished |
| Body change | Libido peaks | Fluid retention | Dryness: eyes, mouth, nose, vagina | Dry vagina |
| Emotional turmoil | "Other" directed: family and career | Sore breasts | —Cessation of menses— | Burning, itchy vulva |
| | Birth control | Pain with intercourse | Pain with intercourse | Urethritis and cystitis |
| | | Aches and pains | Decreased libido | Vaginitis |
| | | Tricky gut | Dizziness | Stress incontinence |
| | | Migraines | Migraines | Hypertension |
| | | Sleep disruption | Sleep disorder | Bone pain |
| | | | Fatigue | Fractures |
| | | | Achiness | Foot and leg cramps |

| | | | | |
|---|---|---|---|---|
| WHO AM I? | I AM FUNCTIONING! | Fatigue | Formication | Joint and muscle aches |
| What's happening to my body? | I have jobs. | Decreasing short-term memory | Decreased short-term memory | Wrinkles and droops |
| I'm changing. | People depend on me. | | Emotional extremes: depression, sadness and grief, apathy, rage, intolerance | Memory improved |
| I am so alone. | | | | Emotional stability |
| | | | | |
| WHO AM I? | | WHO AM I? | WHERE AM I HEADING? | I AM ME AND I AM HERE! |
| What's happening to my body? | | What's happening to my body? | I am out of control. | I am centered. |
| I'm changing. | | I'm changing. | My perceptions and values are shifting. | I am present. |
| I am so alone. | | I am so alone. | I am so alone. | I am unique, part of all. |
| | | | | I am free. |

description of symptoms triggers an insight, as it did when ChaiChin came in for her annual Pap smear. Like so many of my patients, ChaiChin is a dynamite woman. She's a special education teacher who is very involved and active in her community. Like me, she had her children at a later than ususal age, and she was now forty-three years old with a three-year-old daughter. When I mentioned that short-term memory problems go with the whole hormonal process of perimenopause, she grabbed my arm and said, "Michele! I thought I had early Alzheimer's, but I was too afraid to mention it! I've known for weeks that I had this appointment, but I almost had to cancel because I forgot to make child-care arrangements for Betsy!"

Marty put it pretty plainly: "I don't mind the reading glasses, the elastic waistbands, the orthotics in my wider shoes," she said, "but I do really miss my mind. I now make lists to remind myself to check my other lists."

Weight gain usually begins in the perimenopausal phase, and by the end of the menopause the average woman has gained twelve pounds. Most women, including me, absolutely hate this and complain bitterly about the near impossibility of losing the extra pounds. Having become philosophical after my own battle of the bulge, I point out that this is Nature's way of giving women a reservoir of estrogen, stored in their body fat, perhaps to ease some of the symptoms of transition from menstruating woman to postmenopausal woman, from matron to crone. Somewhere along the line, an analogy with pregnancy came to my mind: to me, it seems as if perimenopause is a time of conception and gestation of the next half of our lives; like pregnancy, perimenopause is a time of being aware of bodily changes, of changing self-image, and, at times, of feeling out of control. There is a physiological inevitability to this whole process, but it can be a time of exciting psycho-spiritual growth and change.

It took me a while to put two and two together when it came to the complaints I was hearing from women who said they felt angry and fed up and generally had less tolerance for situations, people, and behaviors than they had had in the past. Finally, sheer repetition made me hear and understand the connection between the psychological distress I was hearing about and the physical complaints being described by the same women. What I think is that at this time in our lives, when physical and emotional changes are going on, there is also an impetus to change our domestic lives, our work lives, our social lives, and maybe also society. Most of the impetus for change is good, but sometimes the baby is thrown out with the bath water. Or, more often, the husband.

My friend Myra is currently in this stage, manifesting rage at her husband for his lifelong trait of lack of assertiveness. Theirs is a good marriage, but lately she has been wondering if she can continue to live with this man. Her women friends listen sympathetically and suggest she wait a few months before seeing a lawyer.

Gail, on the other hand, endured twenty years of an abusive marriage to an alcoholic. She was the woman who "walked into doors" and "fell down stairs"—and every other socially acceptable excuse for injuries. One night, as she lay awake, flashing, she had the sudden realization that this was an intolerable situation that would never change, and in the morning, after her husband had gone to work, Gail packed and left. Today she is a full-time college student, and she hopes to become a drug and alcohol rehabilitation counselor.

*Tricky gut* is the term I've come to use for a catch-all of irritable bowel–like symptoms or food intolerance symptoms that many women begin to experience in their forties, together with other aches and pains. Sometimes, as migraines often do, these symptoms wax and wane with the hormonal cycles. But in some women they seem to have no pattern. A premenstrual stress chart (PMS chart) like the one on pages 10 and 11 is very helpful in tracking patterns of distress associated with a woman's hormonal fluctuations. Needless to say, a visit to a doctor is necessary to make sure that the symptoms are not being caused by a stomach or an intestinal disease or disorder.

As my patients approach menopause, often the first symptoms they tell me about are difficulty with intercourse, sleep difficulties, and short-term memory problems. Many of my patients have already discussed their vaginal symptoms with their primary health care provider and have been told that the vagina is fine: adequate moisture, no sign of infection, and so on. All this can be perfectly true, but a woman may still experience the dry, burning sensation that characteristically comes later, with atrophic vaginitis. (*Atrophic vaginitis* is a condition of the vagina in which the vaginal walls become thin because of lack of estrogen. The symptoms are tenderness and itching.) If a culture for beta streptococcal infection has not been taken, my first step is to take a culture, just to be sure, because beta or b-strep infection can cause these symptoms. Most of the time, however, the symptoms really are just a "developmental milestone."

And many women, even while they complain about sleep problems and short-term memory difficulties, try to "explain the problems away": "I just have too many things on my mind," they say, or "I lie awake and work on all my leftover issues from the day." These tribulations may visit a woman as early as her mid-forties, even occasionally her late thirties, and as late as her early fifties. Being aware of perimenopausal symptoms may help them get some relief, an understanding ear, or at least reassurance that these problems are part of a natural process.

## *Menopause*

At menopause, symptoms become most noticeable and troublesome. For many women this phase can mean a descent into the pit or, viewed differently, into the dark, close tunnel of the birth canal, feeling squeezed on all sides, isolated, alone, and struggling. A woman can feel totally out of control and unable to regain control. For many of us, this is a time of simplification in our lives—ridding ourselves of "excess baggage."

Nora is a psychologist with a thriving practice and a university teaching position. She is divorced with grown children and, until two years ago, enjoyed her comfortable social life in a Washington, D.C., suburb. Two years ago, subtle changes began in her body and, at the same time, as she says, she began shedding. "First it was a lot of old stuff that had been hanging around for years, then clothes that I hadn't worn in a couple of years. Finally, I decided anything I hadn't used in two years could go, and then I found myself putting my house on the market. It sold and now I rent a room and everything I own fits in my car. I'm thinking of moving to Idaho."

For me, simplifying meant dropping memberships in medical societies or associations that were mostly "old boy" networks and joining more women's organizations on a business and professional level. It was a time of beginning to say no instead of soldiering on, doing everything I was asked to do.

Actually, I only developed my healthy instinct after exploring the bottom of the pit. This happened during the summer—a typical New England summer with relatively hot days and cold nights. In mid-June, I found myself shedding my

*PMS Chart*

INSTRUCTIONS: For each day of the month,
1. Use the small box on the left to chart the days you are menstruating with a red M. If there is spotting or very light flow, chart with a small s.
2. Use the middle box to chart your three main symptoms. Identify them by the first letter. For example: anger = A, depression = D, migraine = M. To distinguish variations in severity, it is helpful to use small letters on a mild day and capital letters for a bad day. Depression on a mild day = d; on a bad day = D. Chart any day you have menstrual cramps with a C.
3. Weigh first thing in the morning and insert your weight in the box on the right.

Source: Modified from "Chart for Premenstrual Syndrome," PMS/ACT, 722 Route 3a, Bldg. 2, Suite 13, Bow, NH 03304. Nyla D. Hiltz, R.N.

|  |  | Month 1 |  |
| --- | --- | --- | --- |
| *Day of the Month* | *M or s?* | *Symptoms* | *Weight* |
| 1 |  |  |  |
| 2 |  |  |  |
| 3 |  |  |  |
| 4 |  |  |  |
| 5 |  |  |  |
| 6 |  |  |  |
| 7 |  |  |  |
| 8 |  |  |  |
| 9 |  |  |  |
| 10 |  |  |  |
| 11 |  |  |  |
| 12 |  |  |  |
| 13 |  |  |  |
| 14 |  |  |  |
| 15 |  |  |  |
| 16 |  |  |  |
| 17 |  |  |  |
| 18 |  |  |  |
| 19 |  |  |  |
| 20 |  |  |  |
| 21 |  |  |  |
| 22 |  |  |  |
| 23 |  |  |  |
| 24 |  |  |  |
| 25 |  |  |  |
| 26 |  |  |  |
| 27 |  |  |  |
| 28 |  |  |  |
| 29 |  |  |  |
| 30 |  |  |  |
| 31 |  |  |  |

| | Month 2 | | | | Month 3 | |
|---|---|---|---|---|---|---|
| M or s? | Symptoms | Weight | | M or s? | Symptoms | Weight |
| | | | | | | |
| | | | | | | |
| | | | | | | |
| | | | | | | |
| | | | | | | |
| | | | | | | |
| | | | | | | |
| | | | | | | |
| | | | | | | |
| | | | | | | |
| | | | | | | |
| | | | | | | |
| | | | | | | |
| | | | | | | |
| | | | | | | |
| | | | | | | |
| | | | | | | |
| | | | | | | |
| | | | | | | |
| | | | | | | |
| | | | | | | |
| | | | | | | |
| | | | | | | |
| | | | | | | |
| | | | | | | |
| | | | | | | |
| | | | | | | |
| | | | | | | |
| | | | | | | |
| | | | | | | |
| | | | | | | |
| | | | | | | |
| | | | | | | |

usual nighttime flannels for a light cotton nightie. Then the covering sheet went, too. Finally, I set up a fan to blow directly on me, but still I couldn't sleep! Or, to be more precise, I was awake for fifteen to twenty minutes every hour! By late July, I was exhausted and unable to cope. I decided to take charge when I found myself weeping over my son's cat, Velcro, murmuring that Velcro was the only one who loved me!

Georgia came in the office to ask about her eyes. She stated that maybe she should have seen her optometrist but was afraid that something more general might be wrong, such as diabetes or allergies or some skin problem with the inside of her lids. The problem was that she could no longer tolerate wearing her contact lenses. I asked her a series of questions, including a checklist of menopausal symptoms. She did not have any symptoms related to diabetes or allergy, but she was having pain with attempted intercourse and had little interest in sex, although she has an exceptionally close relationship with her husband. She was having bad night sweats and wasn't able to sleep beyond 5 A.M., and her periods were totally unpredictable, ranging from every two weeks to every two months. Examination confirmed what I'd already guessed: her contact lens difficulty was due to dry eyes. The vagina is not the only moist area that gets dry due to lack of estrogen; it happens in the mouth, nose, and eyes, as well.

One odd symptom of menopause deserves special notice. *Formication* is an itchy sensation that feels like insects are crawling on the skin. It is not the most common menopausal symptom, but as many as 10 percent of women may experience it. Most commonly, the sensation occurs in only one or two areas, and there is no rash, redness, or other visible sign on the skin. Women who experience formication of course want an explanation for this odd sensation. In desperation, women sometimes go to be checked for scabies, skin cancer, or other disorders. Mary, for example, was convinced she had hookworm, while Wendy was sure that the sensation was caused by a homeopathic remedy she had taken five years previously. In menopausal women, formication is most often caused by the same thing that causes other physical symptoms: hormonal imbalance. (See Chapter 5 for more information about this symptom.)

Funmi and Gratia are both women who had very active sexual lives and strong libidos. Suddenly, at age forty-five for Funmi and fifty-one for Gratia, they found that they couldn't care less. Funmi shocked herself by saying to her husband, "Again, honey? We just did it last month." Gratia was afraid of losing her husband, who is a decade younger than she is. Pain was not the problem for Funmi or for Gratia, as they had both retained adequate moisture.

The popular media contribute to the image that the older woman can be even sexier than she was in her thirties. For some this may be true, but most of the women I've talked with experience a decrease in sexual desire and a decrease in intensity of orgasm. Some actually go through a phase of finding sexual intimacy repugnant, and this seems to hold true in lesbian as well as in heterosexual relationships. Most women enjoy the cuddling and closeness and would be satisfied with that, while some experience grief and a sense of lost vitality and spark in life, and others feel that their relationships are jeopardized. As a rule, I encourage women to view this time not as a loss of physical relationship with others, but as a broadening sensuality that is not as focused on the sexual. For me, this has expressed itself as a decision to wear jewel-like colors and soft textures, to enjoy the smell of the wind, damp soil, oranges. To enjoy the silkiness of my husband's skin, the softness of my daughter's hair, and the amber depths of my son's eyes—the aesthetic appreciation of bodies and faces.

As women, we are accustomed to cycles and seasons, but the crossing of the threshold of menopause into autumn brings grief, rage, fear, and great sadness to many women. Have you ever on a luminous autumn day had a shiver of anticipation of winter to come? And felt regret at the passing of the summer flowers and warmth? You might forget at that moment about the different pleasures of winter, and that spring and autumn come again, and that the seeds lying dormant or started in winter burst forth in glory come spring.

The fear of mortality may become a great issue, more so for women recently bereaved, especially by the death of a husband or mother. Each of us needs, in her own way, to accept mortality. Talking with a spiritual counselor can be of tremendous value.

One sign of the fear of our own mortality may be the fear of physically aging—of becoming wrinkled, with skin droops, age spots, gray hair; of being fat or scrawny and shrunken; of becoming invisible. I am reminded of an anecdote told by my brother about his attendance at a high-powered computer systems workshop. "Do you know, we were sitting there and a dumpy little woman in about her mid-fifties, with salt and pepper hair and wearing some sort of jogging outfit, stepped to the podium. I was stunned, but she turned out to be the best speaker there and really knew her stuff." My brother's excitement at hearing a very well regarded expert speak knowledgeably about her subject overcame his initial impression of the speaker's physical presentation.

We women have internalized much of this unconscious sexism and ageism. We fear the loss of sexual appeal as perceived by our society and fail to realize that charisma and magnetism have little to do with age. Somehow, we fail to notice that many of the very attractive women we see are undeniably in our age group.

Some women have defined themselves as "mother" and feel a loss of sense of purpose and meaning as the end of child-bearing approaches. The "empty nest" days are upon us, and with the empty nest comes a large void. Or, a woman may be in a new relationship and wish to have a child with her new partner but finds that it isn't possible. Or menopause occurs too young, either prematurely or surgically.

Two nights ago, in my office during a joint conference with her husband, Gina put many of these changes in a positive framework: "This is my time. Always before it's been time for you [her husband] or the kids or my parents . . . or any of a million other things. But this is my time to find *me* again and learn a new reality and new ways to be creative. I need your acceptance and support. But, please, don't try to *fix* me—I'm not broken."

## Postmenopause

For most women the postmenopausal phase is a time of quiet after the storm, of turbulence remembered in stillness. Most of the women I know, after going through the whole meno-pausal experience with some degree of consciousness and re-flection, are grateful to be at this point and are aware of a flowering of possibilities.

Letitia, at age seventy, went back to school and earned a de-gree in philosophy, saying, "This is just for me and I am loving every minute of it!" Sara, at fifty-one, is making the transition from schoolteacher to documentary filmmaker. Chamique and Kathryn are enjoying the closeness of early retirement with their best friends—their spouses! Eileen now teaches yoga, after thirty years of hospital nursing. Denise, a psychia-trist, has semiretired to teach voice lessons. Dolly, a lawyer for the past twenty-five years, is now a contemplative nun. Jean, a college professor, has become a recognized and published expert on ecologically sustainable communities. The common experience of inner freedom, a sense of their own uniqueness, and the value of their contribution as role models has allowed these women to mature and age gracefully. They are powerful women, as are you and I.

For many of us today—the war babies and the baby boomers—the practical side of life remains difficult. We are still raising teen-age children and at the same time caring for aging parents. Our contributions as care providers should not be minimized. Indeed, most women are unsung heroines. I applaud us all.

For the majority of women, hot flashes and night sweats stop within two years of the last period. For probably less than 2 percent of women, however, they continue indefinitely.

On the more mundane side, fine creations do require more care as time passes, and this is a phase of revisiting health risk assessments periodically (at least every five years) and making sure that our initial management choices are choices that we would still choose. If not, it's time to revise them.

# CHAPTER 2

# Health Concerns Now
## Cardiovascular Disease, Osteoporosis, and Endometrial and Breast Cancer

Most of us fear breast cancer. This is a fact that is given much coverage in the press and in our collective psyche. We think of scheduling our yearly exam to have our breasts checked and to have a Pap smear. Many women see the "to hormone or not to hormone" question solely in terms of its effect on the risks of breast cancer. How realistic is this? Here are some other facts:

*Fact:* More women have died from lung cancer in recent years than from breast cancer. Seventy-five percent of these deaths are directly attributable to tobacco smoking. *"You've come a long way, baby."*

*Fact:* More than half of the deaths in women over age fifty are due to cardiovascular disease, including heart attacks, strokes, and congestive heart failure. *Cardiovascular disease is the number-one killer of American women.*

*Fact:* Slightly more women than men develop cancer of the colon each year. Colon cancer is the third leading cause of death in women in the United States.

*Fact:* Average bone loss in women by age seventy is 40 percent, and a great many women suffer from the pain, cost, and decreased quality of life that accompanies osteoporosis.

We must be aware of our risks in a realistic way and assess them early enough to affect the outcomes. Although women make more patient visits to medical facilities than men, many of our preventive care needs are not adequately addressed. In fact, it would too often seem that we are viewed as reproductive and psychiatric "units." Certainly that is the implication of a recent Continuing Medical Education session on women's health to which I was invited. The topics discussed were Breast Cancer: New Approaches to Diagnosis; Hormone Replacement Therapy; Depression and Anxiety in the Menopausal Years; and New Pharmacologic Agents for Treating Depression. I have to ask: This is women's *health?*

Perimenopause is an ideal time to obtain a health risk assessment from your health care provider, including the usual breast and pelvic exams and Pap smear, along with

- a complete blood count,
- blood chemistries, including cholesterol, triglycerides, HDL and LDL, TSH,* and serum iron, and
- a discussion of lifestyle factors such as diet, exercise, smoking, and alcohol intake.

Exploring the advisability of having mammography and bone densitometry studies also makes sense at this time. A body composition measurement by bioimpedance may also be helpful. Family risk factors should be discussed and should become part of an ongoing consideration of risk and treatment. If you are forty-five or older, I would strongly urge you to have a bone density study, a screen for colorectal cancer, and a mammogram. These are all parts of a fact-finding mis-

*HDL = high-density lipoproteins (the so-called good cholesterol, which apparently has a protective effect in relation to atherosclerosis); LDL = low-density lipoproteins (the so-called bad cholesterol; desirable levels are below 130 mg/dl); TSH = thyroid-stimulating hormone. Cholesterol is a fat that, when elevated, can significantly increase the risk of heart attack and stroke. Triglycerides are fats that also are heart unhealthy when elevated and are significant indicators of diabetes risk. Diabetes also increases the risk of heart attack.

sion in which we obtain information useful to our overall purpose of maintaining good health as we age.

Ruth is a good example of a person who benefited from this approach. She is a housewife and mother of two teenagers and was feeling very well until sometime in 1995, when she began to have a lot of trouble with constipation. At her yearly exam, a blood test showed a higher cholesterol level than she'd ever had, and her doctor suggested adding more fiber to her diet and adding exercise to her daily routine. Over the next six months, she began to gain weight, feel depressed and sluggish, and have trouble with short-term memory. None of the symptoms was severe or dramatic, but the overall effect was decreasing her enjoyment of life and effectiveness in her family. She was tempted to chalk it up to her age but decided to talk with me about it first. As it turned out, her thyroid-stimulating hormone (TSH) was elevated, indicating that her thyroid hormone levels were *low*. Treatment with thyroid hormone quickly restored Ruth's zest for life. It's worth noting that as many as 17 percent of women (the proportion increases with age) have thyroid failure, and, although their symptoms may be mild, this condition increases their cardiovascular risk and may increase their risk of developing colorectal cancer.

Serum iron should be checked simply because so many women supplement their dietary iron intake, and too much is as bad as too little.

## Cardiovascular Disease

Although heart disease has been known to be the number-one killer of American women since 1908, somehow we continue to think of heart disease primarily as a man's disease. In fact, since 1991, more women than men have died of this disease.

- In 1993, cardiovascular disease accounted for 45 percent of all deaths in women, compared with 39 percent in men.
- In 1993, twice as many women died of heart disease as died from all forms of cancer combined.
- More than 50 percent of women over age sixty-five have high blood pressure, and 33 percent of women over age sixty-five have some form of coronary artery disease. Between the ages of forty-five and sixty-four, this figure is greater than 10 percent, comparable with the lifetime risk of breast cancer.
- Black women are 70 percent more likely to die of heart disease than white women.

Even though these statistics should mean that cardiovascular disease, stroke, and heart attack ought to be concerns for all women and their doctors, the sad truth is that women are less likely than men to be promptly diagnosed with heart disease and, when diagnosed, are less likely to receive aggressive treatment.

Risk factors for cardiovascular disease for men and women are very similar: smoking, high blood pressure, lack of exercise, obesity, and family history. But heart disease appears about ten years later in women and is often compounded by diabetes and abnormal blood fats. In women, high triglycerides and low HDL are more accurate predictors of coronary heart disease than in men, and the significance of LDL is less certain. Being postmenopausal for any reason—naturally, surgically, or through illness—is a major risk factor.

A woman with coronary artery disease may not have the symptoms we probably think of when we think of angina or heart attack. Yes, she may have classic chest pain with left arm radiation, brought on by exercise and relieved by rest, but for the older woman, shortness of breath, fatigue, "indigestion," or a general feeling of "being sick" may be subtle signs of heart disease. Also, chest pain may occur even when she is resting, and may be different from the classic chest pain.

Unfortunately, we do not have enough studies on women and heart disease to give definitive advice. For example, lowering high blood pressure has had disappointing results—it doesn't seem to benefit women as much as we might expect. It is encouraging that in 1995 the National Institutes of Health allocated 16 percent of its cardiovascular disease research budget to research specifically addressing the disease in women, although this still seems a small amount, considering the proportion of women in the population.

Recently women have asked me about the reports that HRT increases risk in women with existing coronary artery disease. These reports are based on the HERS trials, the results of which were published in 1998. This study has been widely criticized in the professional literature, both because there are serious design flaws that interfere with the statistical validity of the data and because the progestin chosen to be used in the study was medroxyprogesterone acetate. As I discuss later in this book, this form of progesterone blocks any beneficial effect of estrogen on cardiovascular risk; this disadvantage of medroxyprogesterone acetate has been widely reported in the literature for many years. Many studies, whether laboratory studies or studies in groups of women, have demonstrated an overall beneficial effect on cardiovascular risk. It is true that in many studies of many therapies—for example, insulin for diabetes and lipid-lowering drugs for cardiovascular events— there is a small increase in adverse events immediately after the therapy is started. This effect is poorly understood and does not negate the long-term benefits of these therapies.

It is clear from recent studies, however, that the use of hormone replacement in women with existing coronary artery disease contributes to a worsening of this disease. We are still left with many paradoxes and unanswered questions, but with what we currently know, we clearly should not look to hormone replacement as a preventive measure for cardiovascular disease.

It would make sense, unless proven otherwise, to assume that the risk factors relevant to men are also risk factors for us. Certainly the following are all good prescriptions for our general health as well as our cardiovascular health:

- Refrain from smoking.
- Eat a healthful diet containing lots of fruit, vegetables, and whole grains.
- Maintain our bodies at 18 to 26 percent fat.
- Exercise on a regular basis.
- Enjoy restful sleep.

See Appendix 1 for a couple of healthful dieting plans to both reduce blood fats and lose weight.

Garlic in a dose of 300 mg (milligrams) three times daily, containing 1.3 percent allium per dose, has been shown in several studies to lower total cholesterol and triglycerides. A recent study found that a diet low on the glycemic index (see Appendix 1) will raise HDL, especially in women. I had a mixture of amino acids, vitamins, and minerals compounded for my patients and advised them to take three doses daily. This mixture—of 333 mg carnitine, 250 mg folic acid, 50 mg pantothenic acid, and 25 mg chromium GTF—has helped my patients who were unable to lower their lipids by diet alone. Also, gugulipid, an Ayurvedic herbal preparation, in a dose standardized to contain 25 mg of gugulsterones, taken three times daily, has been shown to lower the level of low-density lipoproteins ("bad" cholesterol). (*Ayurvedic* is traditional Hindu medicine; *gugulsterones* is the active chemical in *gugulipid*.)

## Osteoporosis

Osteoporosis, or thinning of the bones, is a silent process that is too often not recognized until a woman has lost significant height or has fractured a bone. Previous generations have been relatively helpless to prevent or treat this problem, but this is no longer true. The woman at greatest risk has been characterized as having the following characteristics:

* fair hair and complexion
* of Northern European descent
* sedentary
* slight of build
* has borne and nursed children
* a family history of osteoporosis.

Additional risk factors for developing osteoporosis are smoking, insufficient calcium intake, excessive alcohol consumption, use of cortisone or prednisone, hyperthyroidism, and any eating disorder.

Like most physicians, I used to use these guidelines almost exclusively to discuss risk of osteoporosis with women. No longer! Lee converted me to being a true believer in routine bone densities (densitometry). Lee, two years postmenopausal, had been a teacher of martial arts for the past twenty years, had never been pregnant, never smoked or drank, followed an excellent diet, had a strong and muscular build, and, aside from an occasional cold, had never been ill. Nor did she use any medications. Her only risk factors were that she is blond and of Northern European descent. But, consistent with her proactive approach to health, Lee wanted a bone density study. So, it was arranged. And, much to my horror and amazement, Lee was already osteoporotic! This was an eye-opener for both of us and led to my routine recommendation of bone densities for women and to Lee's decision to use hormone replacement therapy, which she would not otherwise have considered.

Osteoporosis may not kill us in the numbers that coronary heart disease does, but it does cause much grief and disability. One out of two women age fifty and over will suffer a broken bone caused by osteoporosis. In a woman with osteoporosis, fractures can result from very minor traumas or even simple everyday activities. My sister hugged our mother and broke Mom's rib. Suma sneezed and a vertebra collapsed. Not only is there a cost in terms of chronic pain, hospitalizations, and deaths from fractures, but there is also loss of independence and dignity when a person is forced to curtail activities because she is frail.

We all need to be aware that osteoporosis can be prevented and treated. As with most other health issues, the first step is a realistic risk assessment. At least 30 percent of your bone mass must already have been lost before a diagnosis of osteoporosis can be made by standard X-ray. And once that much bone mass is lost, it's very late to begin treatment. For this reason, I suggest that all menopausal women have a bone densitometry done. This is very important timing, because in the first years after menstruation ceases, bone loss accelerates to two to four times the premenopausal rate. In some women this rapid loss continues. For follow-up, I like to repeat the bone density in three to five years, depending on the initial report.

If bone loss shows up on the bone densitometry, I often will follow-up one year later by doing an Ntx urine test, which measures the end products of bone turnover. This study, rather than telling us how dense a woman's bones are, tells us how rapidly she is breaking down bone. Here in New Hampshire, the average cost of the bone density test is around $250, and a woman should plan ahead to pay for it out of pocket, since many but not all insurers will cover the study. Recently, a new methodology was approved which uses an ultrasound of the heel. This test is less expensive and is an acceptable screen.

*"If my bones are okay, what should I do to prevent osteoporosis?"* Ideally, prevention would begin when we are little girls, with diets high in calcium-rich foods, lots of "sun-safe" exposure to sunshine, and weight-bearing exercise. Another suggestion is to start girls on 600 mg of supplemental calcium when they are about sixteen. I started giving my daughter these supplements when she was in junior high school.

Although we are no longer little girls, a calcium-rich prescription for prevention applies to us, too. Calcium-rich foods include dairy foods, calcium-fortified orange juice, broccoli, deep-green leafies (like kale and dandelion), tofu, and fortified breads and cereals. Calcium-rich herbs include alfalfa, nettle, oat straw, kelp, horsetail, and sage.

Calcium supplements can also be taken by adult women. I often suggest 1500 mg calcium and 750 mg magnesium in combination. (We need magnesium to properly use calcium in our bodies.) I have also observed that a significant number of us have trouble with calcium supplements—our guts don't like them. My suggestion is to keep trying different types of calcium until you find one that doesn't bother you. Very few people are unable to tolerate *all* forms of calcium supplements. It is also important to get 400 IU (international units) of vitamin D and half an hour of sunshine daily.

One of my patients remarked about her bones that "if you don't abuse them, you lose them." This is going a bit far, but you do need to stress your bones by doing weight-bearing exercise on a regular basis. Swimming just doesn't do it. Walking is a safe weight-bearing exercise and is the most popular form of exercise for women.

*"What if my bones aren't so good? What do I do now?"* The first choice for many in treating osteoporosis is hormone replacement therapy, which is also good osteoporosis *preventive* medicine for many women. Estrogen offers effective protection and, of the osteoporosis treatments available, probably has the least objectionable side effects. To remineralize bone that has already started to become thin, I suggest taking calcium hydroxyapatite with boron as perhaps the best form of calcium for this purpose.

We now also have several drugs available to treat osteoporosis. Micalcin, Fosamax, and Actonel have recently received FDA approval for this purpose. Didronel is another drug that has been used to treat osteoporosis for several years, although it doesn't have FDA approval for this purpose.

Micalcin is a nasal spray taken as one squirt in a nostril daily. It has been demonstrated to increase bone mass at a rate of approximately 3 percent over a three-year period and to decrease vertebral fracture rates by 30 percent over a three-year period. Technically speaking, Micalcin has been around for a long time and, technically speaking, is not a drug—it is the hormone calcitonin. Until Micalcin became available, however, calcitonin had to be administered by very painful injections. Unfortunately, Micalcin has not proven to be as good as other drugs for treating postmenopausal osteoporosis.

Didronel is approved in many European countries for the treatment of osteoporosis and has been available for more than ten years. It is dosed on an intermittent schedule of 400 mg daily for two weeks every three months (for example, the first two weeks of December, March, June, and September). It has been shown to increase spinal bone density about

5 percent and hip density about 3 percent over five years. Didronel must be taken one hour before or two hours after a meal.

Fosamax was the first nonhormonal approach to treatment of osteoporosis approved in this country. It has been shown to increase bone mass 7 to 8 percent over a three-year period and to significantly decrease fracture rates. In fact, we now know that Fosamax can decrease the occurrence of new fractures by as much as 50 percent three years after treatment begins. An increase in bone density can be seen as early as three months after beginning Fosamax.

Fosamax must be taken according to very specific instructions: you must take it first thing in the morning, with only plain water, on an empty stomach. You must not lie down again or eat or drink anything else for a minimum of thirty minutes (two hours is optimal). Food and beverages other than water can interfere with the absorption of Fosamax and therefore can make treatment less effective. Lying down can greatly increase the risk of gastrointestinal esophageal reflux (GERD, formerly known as heartburn) and irritation or erosion of the esophagus. Stomach pain and other gastrointestinal symptoms are the most commonly experienced side effects, although Fosamax is generally well tolerated. One dear relative, of both advanced age and osteoporosis, decided that Fosamax was not the answer for her because it so disturbed the lovely morning ritual of tea, reading, and conversation in bed with her husband.

Actonel is a kissing cousin of Fosamax, and is used in exactly the same way as Fosamax. It is somewhat better tolerated than Fosamax. Since we are now able to dose both Fosamax and Actonel with one large dose given on one day each week, the previous disadvantages of taking the drug in such a careful manner, as well as the upset tummy it causes, have been much

**Table 2. Health Concerns Raised Now**

| Concern | Symptoms | Diagnostic Tests | Prevention | Treatment |
|---|---|---|---|---|
| Hypothyroidism | weight gain<br>depression<br>sluggishness<br>memory problems | TSH | | thyroid-hormone |
| Cardiovascular<br>disease | high blood pressure<br>chest pain<br>shortness of breath<br>fatigue<br>"indigestion" | blood fat profile<br>stress test | exercise<br>no smoking<br>herbs<br>medication | *same as for prevention* |
| Osteoporosis | loss of height<br>fractures | awareness of risk<br>factors<br>bone densitometry | diet<br>exercise<br>no smoking | estrogens, progestins,<br>and androgens<br>Fosamax<br>HCTZ |

| | | Ntx urine test | supplements: calcium, magnesium, and vitamin D<br>hormones | Didronel<br>Micalcin<br>Evista |
|---|---|---|---|---|
| Endometrial cancer | abnormal bleeding | transvaginal ultrasound<br>endometrial biopsy<br>dilatation and curettage | progesterone | surgery<br>radiation |
| Breast cancer | | monthly self-exam<br>mammography<br>professional exam<br>ultrasound<br>needle aspiration<br>biopsy | no smoking<br>diet (soy)<br>exercise<br>reduce body fat<br>antioxidants<br>? estriol<br>? flax<br>? Tamoxifen | |

diminished. Now, very few women are not able to tolerate one of these drugs.

Other drugs are being developed and tests are being performed on one drug that may need to be administered only once yearly. It is too soon to report much more than this.

Also of interest is that hydrochlorothiazide, or HCTZ, a commonly used blood pressure drug and diuretic, prevents bone loss. As with the other drugs, the protective benefit is lost when you stop taking it. It is by far the cheapest drug alternative we have.

In February 1998 Evista, the first selective estrogen receptor modulator (SERM), was put on the market. This is the first of this class of drugs, offspring of Tamoxifen (an antiestrogen and anticancer drug), but undoubtedly will not be the last. Evista has the FDA nod for the prevention of osteoporosis in high-risk postmenopausal women who either cannot or will not use estrogen. It is hoped that these drugs will also prevent breast cancer. On the face of it these drugs are very promising, but I want to sound a cautionary note: even though in the short term Tamoxifen was not shown to cause endometrial proliferation (see below), ultimately Tamoxifen was demonstrated to pose an increased risk for endometrial cancer. So far, only studies of short-term use of Evista are available, and they show no endometrial proliferation as a result of taking Evista in the short term. Again, however, long-term studies have not yet been done. Also, the question has not yet been satisfactorily answered as to whether the breast cancer data represent a true preventive benefit or just a delay in onset. Only time will answer these questions. Other potential side effects of Evista are unwanted hot flashes and vaginal dryness.

A number of other drugs for osteoporosis are in various stages of research. The Women's Health Equity Act has taken on responsibility for seeking increased research funding for this and other important women's health issues. As individuals, our responsibility is to assess our risks early and put preventive measures in place. We should then periodically reassess our risks and the preventive or treatment measures we have in place, to be sure we've made the choices that are effective for us as individuals. (For more information, see "Fractures and Bone Pain" in Chapter 6.)

## Endometrial Cancer

Endometrial cancer is cancer of the lining of the uterus. This cancer accounts for less than 1 percent of deaths in American women, but it's an important issue to address in a book about menopause, because the predominant forms of estrogen used as hormone replacement in the United States—estrone and estradiol—cause endometrial cancer in 12 percent of the women using them. This risk is totally negated by using progesterone together with these estrogens. It is this combination of estrogen and progesterone that is commonly referred to as *hormone replacement therapy*, or *HRT*.

The most common symptom of endometrial cancer is abnormal bleeding. Any bleeding after menopause is abnormal. In perimenopause, bleeding too much or too frequently deserves a consult with your doctor. Don't panic, but do check it out. Uncommonly, a postmenopausal woman will have endometrial cells on her Pap smear. This, too, is a reason for your doctor to check further. After all, you're not even supposed to be making the endometrial lining anymore, so why are there cells from the lining on a Pap smear?

The gold standard in investigating abnormal bleeding is an *endometrial biopsy*. (The *gold standard* is the most definitive diagnostic technique available, as accepted by most experts.) In this procedure, a very thin plastic cannula, or tube, is passed into the uterus through the cervical opening. Fragments of endometrial tissue are sucked out through this tube into a collection receptacle, and these cells are then examined for cancerous or precancerous changes.

Gaining increased acceptance for diagnostic purposes is the use of transvaginal ultrasound to measure the thickness of the lining of the uterus. In transvaginal ultrasound, a condom-covered probe is inserted in the vagina; the probe emits high-frequency waves and produces images (on a computer screen) from reflections of those waves. This allows the radiologist or technician to "see" and measure internal organs. The procedure is usually painless. If the thickness exceeds four millimeters, then an endometrial biopsy or a D&C (dilatation and curettage of the uterus) should be done. Ultrasound is less invasive than an endometrial biopsy or a D&C and has increased women's options. It has been made possible by advances in ultrasound technology and advances in the reading of ultrasounds. Remember, though, that these are diagnostic procedures, not treatments.

Hysterosonography is rapidly becoming the gold standard for evaluating bleeding around or after the time of menopause. In this procedure, a contrast medium is instilled in the uterus so that small fibroids or other irregular areas show up better on ultrasound.

## Breast Cancer

But to return to the beginning of this chapter: Breast cancer is the illness most women fear. We march for breast cancer awareness and wear ribbons signifying our desire to overcome this dreaded killer. It accounts for 4 percent of our deaths per year. (Why do we not march for awareness of our vulnerability to heart disease?)

Recently, in a popular magazine, I read interviews with leading women physicians and was a little surprised that several of them suggested that breast self-exam is of little value and only frightens women. Breast self-exam certainly can be frightening, especially if a woman is uncertain about the significance of what she is feeling. If women are taught self-exam at the time of their first gynecological exam, however, and if it is explained that 85 percent of the lumps found in breasts are benign, I believe self-exam can be of value if a woman checks out any new "lumpiness" that she feels.

Mammography is always a loaded question with my patients. Many are fearful of the procedure itself, and some women do find it painful. I advocate screening mammograms with my patients: two or three spaced out during the forties, and every year or two after age fifty. My one biggest argument for this is that early detection gives one more choice. To me, as to many women, this is important. Also, early detection of breast cancer prolongs life.

As indicated in Table 2, there are additional tests that help us in making an early diagnosis of any breast problems. Ultrasound is increasingly being used to augment mammography, especially to differentiate between cysts and more solid "lumps" in the breast. Very often the combination of mammography and ultrasound can provide the reassurance that a breast finding is not malignant. When there is room for doubt, doctors must continue with diagnostic tests until they are reasonably sure that no malignancy exists.

If the mass appears to be cystic, the next step often is a fine-needle aspiration. This may be done in the doctor's office or may be guided by mammogram. The object is to find out whether any fluid can be aspirated (sucked up) and, if so, whether there are any malignant cells in the fluid. Or, a biopsy may be done. The decision to do a biopsy may be made when no fluid can be extracted during a needle aspiration of what is presumed to be a cyst, or because of other suspicious characteristics on exam or mammogram. Biopsies may be done in the conventional surgical fashion or in the new stereotactic method, in which the biopsies are guided by X-ray and done by a special machine. Either way, a sampling of breast tissue is taken to be examined under the microscope. None of us is eager to undergo any of these procedures, but they may save our life.

Statistically, the use of estrogen at any time in one's life increases somewhat the risk of developing breast cancer. Only one form of estrogen (estriol—see Chapter 7) seems to have no breast cancer risk. Also, our risk increases with each decade of life, much like prostate cancer in men, but the nature of the disease seems to change and often seems much less aggressive in older postmenopausal women. Certainly, it is more amenable to treatment.

We really don't know enough about breast cancer. Survival rates are better for women who have no metastases (spread of cancer beyond the breast) at the time of diagnosis, and this helps make the argument for the self-examination and mammography methods of screening.

How can we prevent breast cancer? We should not smoke, and we should be careful of passive smoking and pesticide exposure. We should ingest no more, for example, than three glasses of wine per week (alcohol interferes with the detoxification of estrogen in the liver) and should try to keep our percentage of body fat between 18 and 26 percent. Our diet should be full of whole grains, fruits, and veggies. A very simple rule is to eat for color: a plate of food with deep green, yellow, orange, and red on it is packed with antioxidants. My special treat is at least one red bell pepper each week. Beautiful food is also healthy food.

Soy is an important component of a diet to prevent breast cancer. There is a much lower breast cancer rate in those cultures eating a diet high in soy protein. It has long been recognized, for example, that Japanese women have a very low breast cancer risk. Certain components in soy, the isoflavones, may affect the hormone receptors in a way that prevents cancer. Certainly it is worth including at least two or three helpings of soy in our diets each week. For women who have little experience of or inclination to cook with tofu, tempeh, or miso, I suggest soy milk, texturized vegetable protein, and soy nuts.

Exercise and meditation are also important, if for no other reason than the positive effects of endorphin release. Depression and breast cancer have been linked in a number of studies. Three to four hours of exercise per week may greatly reduce your risk of developing breast cancer or depression.

I think it is also worthwhile to include ground flax seed in your diet. A study looking at oils in the diets of laboratory mice used in breast cancer studies found that mice eating flax seed oil rejected breast cancer. Okay, so I'm not a mouse. It still won't hurt, and it does benefit me in other ways, providing fiber, essential fatty acids, and other beneficial ingredients.

Antiestrogen drugs that are currently being developed will offer protection against osteoporosis and heart disease and will not increase breast cancer risk. A couple of breast cancer specialists are advocating a controversial approach to cancer prevention: a drug regimen to suppress ovarian hormone production throughout a woman's reproductive years except when she wants to conceive. This is thought to reduce our risks from our own natural levels of hormone.

Obviously, we don't yet have the answers. A common-sense "won't hurt, might help" approach is the best we can do at present.

# CHAPTER 3

# Overview of Therapies
## *Allopathic, Complementary, Herbal, and Homeopathic*

When we speak of therapies or therapeutics for menopausal symptoms, we mean treating women for menopausal symptoms. When it comes to this topic, we must keep uppermost in our minds that menopause is a normal and natural process and that following nature's course can be a perfectly good choice. In my view the two most healing resources available to us are, first, ourselves and, second, the circle of women—a kinship of shared experience which transcends socioeconomic differences, geographic distances, and cultural boundaries.

### *Looking to Ourselves*

An underutilized resource is ourselves—that centered place of inner tranquility accessible by a variety of meditative techniques. These techniques are not difficult, tremendously time-consuming, or expensive, nor do they require adherence to any philosophy or theology. They do require practice and enjoyment. My usual method is to be attentive to my breathing and allow it to slow very rhythmically, and in my inner vision, to watch the darkness turn to purple and white light. On a very busy office day, I use this technique periodically for two to three minutes at a time and feel as refreshed as from a nap.

There were times during my menopausal process when I felt too scattered to center easily and had to find other ways. One that worked very well was sitting comfortably and listening attentively to Gregorian chant; within ten minutes, I would feel like my soul had been washed and the day was again possible. My family learned the sign: if Gregorian chant is playing, give Mom some time and space. Another technique that was useful was visualizing the colors of the rainbow, from red to violet, and then, if necessary, counting down steps of a visualized stairway.

My patient Aislin is a perfectionist with a lot of nervous energy. She became very anxious at the mere suggestion of "doing nothing." A simple prop worked for her, however: she made a Japanese sand garden in a wooden tray, using sand and five pretty pebbles. She raked her garden, using a dessert fork, into pretty wave-like patterns for about fifteen minutes each day. After about three weeks of this, she had the "ah-ha" realization that she was, indeed, experiencing a feeling of calm and refreshment, that she was truly taking a step outside of the daily tensions.

Hazel, a dancer and aerobics instructor, is very kinesthetically oriented. She found that adding Tai chi to her accomplishments also added a new dimension to her inner life. (Tai chi has also been shown to decrease fracture rates in people who are elderly, probably by improving balance. It has even been known to lower high blood pressure.)

A fun and very helpful exercise for tangled emotions is keeping a color journal. This tip was given me by a very dear woman, Sarah Lee Sexton, who has since passed on. Two purchases are necessary: a watercolor notebook and either crayons or colored pencils that can also be brushed with water. Each day you simply draw or paint a page in your journal. The only instruction is to use the color or colors that you feel drawn to on that day. This is a wonderful nonverbal, nonthreatening, absolutely private way to express emotion. It is also fun.

## Support from Other Women

Most of our mothers and grandmothers had a very different lifestyle from ours. Their lives were not free of stress and work, of course, but it does seem that they were able to assert their own rhythm, even if unconsciously. Relaxed interaction and sharing with other women, as well as having access to an extended family, were the norm. These activities did not take their place among dozens of other activities, as they would today, all of them being juggled as priorities seeking attention in a woman's life.

I remember my mother's Home Bureau classes in embroidery (she taught it), the Altar and Rosary Society, and the garden she planted with her friend and neighbor, Peg. And my grandmother's afternoon bridge group. And the ladies gathering over many cups of coffee and the occasional glass of wine. And then I think about what effort it would take to incorporate this into my life, when it takes at least two weeks to synchronize schedules with any of my friends.

This is the time to seek out your own circle of women, at work, in your neighborhood, however it can happen, to tap into shared strength. With them, you can laugh, cry, and otherwise put symptoms—and life—into perspective. You don't need an "expert" for this; you are the expert on your own reality. Two friends, Nina and Hannah, brought together a group of co-workers from the small school where they teach. School is left behind and they are private beings within their group. One of my patients, Sue, gathered a group to sing and chant together. Another patient, Bess, conference calls with her two best friends from high school.

If you are looking for a formal support group, your local providers of women's health care may be helpful, or you can contact the North American Menopause Society at 1-900-

370-NAMS, or visit their website at (www.menopause.org). (Note that the telephone call is a toll call, and you will be charged by the minute.)

## Common-Sense Lifestyle Assists

Charting our cycles (I use a PMS chart like the one in Chapter 1) can help us see hormonal influences affecting how we feel, and this can be very reassuring. You can see that you do not *always* feel angry and depressed. Or you can see that there is a definite pattern for your weight gain or migraines. Seeing patterns can help us to identify effective remedial steps or, at least, help us not to schedule a job interview or major presentation on a "bad hair day."

One thing that can help is exercise, which is very important during all the phases of the "change." My advice is always to find some form of exercise that you like, because then you are more likely to stay with it and to derive all of the benefits from it. Exercise raises endorphin levels, leading to a feeling of greater well-being. It helps us to keep our weight stable and to maintain our muscle mass. The firming action of exercise helps to counterbalance the gravitational pull on our bellies, upper arms, breasts, and other soft parts; not least, exercise helps us stay healthy by raising our good cholesterol, keeping us cardiovascularly fit, and preventing osteoporosis. It also decreases the risk for breast cancer (though we don't know why) and depression. A number of women have told me that exercising half an hour daily has greatly helped their sleep problems.

Needless to say, among the common-sense lifestyle measures you can utilize, diet ranks high. This is the time to learn to eat for health. Many of us, in the effort to keep weight down, eat too little, with long intervals between eating, and rely on nutrient-poor pick-me-ups like caffeine or snacks laden with sugar, fat, and salt. To optimize energy and mood levels, eating small amounts every two to three hours makes sense. Good snacks can be a fruit or vegetable with two to three nuts, a tablespoon of seeds, or a non-fat dairy product.

The Mediterranean diet pyramid (see Appendix 1) may be a good guideline to planning your total daily intake. A quick guide is to make sure your plate of food is very colorful, with deep greens, bright reds, yellows, and orange aesthetically arranged among the beige, white, or brown. The brightly colored foods are nutrient-dense as well as pleasing to the eye. It is worthwhile cultivating a taste for them if you don't already have it.

Let me emphasize that there is payback for a good diet: you really do feel better.

I also suggest taking supplemental calcium and magnesium to help safeguard the bones, and vitamin E if hot flashes are a problem. There is evidence that vitamin E can also help prevent arteriosclerotic plaque from adhering to vessels walls. It's a "won't hurt, might help, why not?" scenario.

Weight gain is so distressing to most of us. Very few of us have the culturally desirable svelte boyish figure to begin with, and now here we are needing elastic waistbands! I'll say again that the average weight gain through menopause is twelve pounds. My advice is not to try hard for weight loss at this time, but rather to stabilize your weight by healthful eating and by exercising. If you want, weight loss can be addressed later, after your rioting hormones have settled down. Rigorous dieting at this time contributes to the effects of yo-yoing hormones and can aggravate a lot of symptoms. It's not a bad idea to have a high-sensitivity test of thyroid-stimulating hormone to determine whether the hormone is at its proper level, just to make sure you are not one of the women who become hypo-thyroid at this stage (hypothyroidism can cause weight gain).

## Allopathic, Complementary, Herbal, and Homeopathic Therapeutics

For your quick ease of reference, at the end of this chapter I have provided a list of the primary problems and approaches to therapy in perimenopause, menopause, and postmeno-pause (see Table 3). Then, in each of the next three chapters, following the same order as the list in the table, I'll discuss the various specific therapeutics for the symptoms. I will describe several approaches to treatment:

1. *Allopathic.* Allopathic medicine is what we think of as regular medical treatment, usually provided by physicians—also called medical doctors—who have been to medical school and hold the M.D. degree.

2. *Complementary.* Complementary or alternative therapies (also called *unconventional* or *unproven therapies*), although they are not scientifically proven, often do provide great re-lief. Alternative medicine includes all nonallopathic therapies, such as homeopathy, acupuncture, and herbs. Complemen-tary medicine is what I practice. I am an allopath (a conven-tional medical doctor) who also includes a variety of alterna-tive modalities in my practice. I choose either by what seems most likely to work best in a particular situation or by the preference of my patient. My overactive curiosity has led me down this path, and my patients have benefited.

3. *Herbal.* Herbal medicine is the tradition upon which much of pharmacology was originally based, and the tradition remains vital today. In the early years of this country, many families maintained medicinal gardens, and every housewife

spent part of her time preparing remedies for family and friends. Ample evidence of this can be seen in old cookbooks. If you are not familiar with herbalism and its terminology, you may find a few definitions helpful. We most commonly think in terms of taking pills and capsules, but herbs are also available in the following forms:

- A *tincture* is an alcohol (or, less commonly, a glycerine) extract of an herb. For example, one might take an ounce of St. John's wort blossoms and pour over them an ounce or two of pure grain alcohol and let the mixture sit for about six weeks. Then it is strained and the strained liquid becomes the tincture. Tinctures are the most potent forms of herbal medicine, but they require commitment on the part of the user, because they do not taste very good.
- A *tea* is made by pouring very hot water over leaves, twigs, roots, or fruits of a plant. Very occasionally a tea can be made by boiling the dried herb in the water. An example of this is sage tea, which is boiled to evaporate toxic materials.
- An *infusion* is made by steeping fresh herb in cold or hot liquid. When you make sun tea, you are making an infusion.

When self-treating with herbals, remember that anything that is potent enough to have a significant beneficial effect may also have potent side effects. Make every effort to educate yourself, and be sure to inform all your health care providers about all the medications you are taking, regardless of whether they are prescription medications or not. Herbs can be very valuable allies, but they must be treated with respect.

4. *Homeopathic.* Although in the following chapters I in-

clude homeopathic remedies for most of the symptoms of perimenopause, menopause, and postmenopause, I am not a homeopath. Having said that I am not a homeopath, I am reminded that many people don't really know what homeopathy is, so let me describe the origins of homeopathic medicine and its principles.

Homeopathy is an approach to treatment founded in the late 1700s by Dr. Samuel Hahnemann. It was a popular form of medicine in the United States for about a hundred years but fell out of favor here early in the twentieth century. In Europe it continued—and continues—to be very popular and, indeed, has been utilized by the royal family of England.

The early homeopaths were all medical doctors, but homeopathy is no longer taught in medical schools or used in hospitals in this country. (Homeopathic hospitals still exist in London and Paris.) In the United States today there is a revival of interest in homeopathy, and many lay practitioners (people without formal medical training or medical degrees) practice homeopathy.

The basic principle of homeopathic prescribing is the Law of Similars, which goes "Let likes be treated with likes." The foundations of this law are the following:

a. The action of a drug can be observed by administering it to a healthy person and then observing and recording the resulting symptoms and objective physical findings. This process is called a *proving.* Example: Arsenic can cause diarrhea.

b. The action of the drug in the healthy person demonstrates the therapeutic action in a sick person. Example: Arsenicum can treat diarrhea. (*Arsenicum* is an extremely diluted form of arsenic.)

c. The remedy will be chosen by a similarity in the disease

process and the "proving" of a drug in a healthy person. The drug that causes a picture most like the signs and symptoms of the illness is the drug of choice. In other words, the prescribed treatment is "The hair of the dog that bit you."

An immediate question almost anyone would ask is, If these remedies cause symptoms in healthy people, won't they poison a sick person? The answer is yes, they would, if they were administered in sufficient amounts, but, in homeopathy, the basic material (again, let's say arsenic) is very much diluted, in a ritual manner called *succussion*. Arsenicum, for example, is arsenic that has been diluted through succussion. It is said that what is active in the remedy is the *essence* of the material. For this reason, it is very unusual for a homeopathic remedy to be poisonous, although there is a potential for this in the case of, for example, arsenic, if even very low potency (3x) arsenicum were given to a child in excess of the labeled recommendations. In the low potencies *homeopathically speaking*, there is less dilution and therefore they are "stronger" in common parlance. (In other words, 3x arsenicum is a stronger dilution of aresenic than 30x arsenicum.)

A paradox in homeopathy is that the more dilute a remedy is, the more potent it is. The remedies that are available over the counter (that is, without a prescription from a homeopathic doctor) are by definition less potent, but they are more concentrated in actual substance. This is confusing at first. The highest potency of any substance available without a prescription is 30x, which means it has been diluted and succussed thirty times.

How do you take these remedies and how are they supplied? Most of them are available as little pellets of lactose (critics say *only* lactose) which you dissolve under the tongue, much as a person takes nitroglycerine. Sometimes they are available in liquid form, as well. There is a cream called Traumeel which my daughter and her fellow dancers say is the best cream for muscle aches.

With this background in place, we can now discuss the various options in relieving menopausal symptoms.

Table 3. *Therapeutic Options in Perimenopause, Menopause, and Postmenopause*

| Problem | Medical | Complementary | Herbal | Homeopathic |
| --- | --- | --- | --- | --- |
| **PERIMENOPAUSE** | | | | |
| Menstural irregularity and PMS | charting | acupuncture | black current seed oil | Belladonna |
| | diagnostic test of endocrine function | charting | black cohosh | charting |
| | diet | diet | borage oil | China |
| | exercise | GLA | cinnamon | Crocus sativa |
| | HRT | ibuprofen | dandelion | Ipecacuanha |
| | ibuprofen | mineral supplements | decrease animal fat | Lachesis |
| | mineral supplements | PMS vitamins | Dong Quai | Natrum mur |
| | NSAIDs | | evening primrose oil | Sabina |
| | oral contraceptives | | flax seed | Secale |
| | PMS vitamins | | hops | Sepia |
| | surgery | | lady's mantle | Sulfur |
| | | | licorice root | |
| | | | pomegranate seeds | |
| | | | raspberry leaf | |

| Aches and pains | | | | |
|---|---|---|---|---|
| diet | acupuncture | borage oil | sage | Arnica |
| drugs | massage | Dong Quai | sarsaparilla | Rhus tox |
| exercise | relaxing | flax seed | shepherd's-purse | |
| vitamin and mineral supplements | therapeutic touch | Kava-Kava | vitex | |
| | | moxibustion | wheat germ oil | |
| | | St. John's wort | wild yam root | |
| | | willow bark | witch hazel | |
| | | | yarrow | |
| | | | yellow dock root | |

**Table 3.** *Therapeutic Options in Perimenopause, Menopause, and Postmenopause* (continued)

| Problem | Medical | Complementary | Herbal | Homeopathic |
|---|---|---|---|---|
| Migraines | charting | acupuncture | black cohosh | Lycopodium |
| | drugs | massage | feverfew | Natrum mur |
| | HRT | therapeutic touch | sage | Pulsatilla |
| | reevaluating self-expectations | | skullcap | Sanguinaria |
| | | | St. John's wort | Silica |
| | | | vervain | Spigelia |
| | | | wild yam | Thuja |
| | | | willow leaf | |
| Decreasing short-term memory | HRT | | black cohosh | Lycopodium |
| | memory exercises | | Dong Quai | |
| | reminders | | Ginko biloba | |
| | | | Ostaderm | |

| | | | | |
|---|---|---|---|---|
| Emotional turmoil | androgens<br>DHEA<br>diet<br>drugs<br>exercise<br>HRT | counseling<br>discuss libido<br>changes<br>educate family<br>journaling<br>massage<br>quiet time<br>rhythm<br>women friends | black cohosh<br>Dong Quai<br>ginseng<br>Kava-Kava<br>liferoot flowers<br>motherwort<br>passion flower<br>sage<br>St. John's wort<br>valerian<br>vitex<br>wild yam | Arsenicum<br>Aurum metallicum<br>Calcarea<br>Calms forte<br>Caulophyllum<br>Cimifuga<br>Natrum mur<br>Phosphorus<br>Pulsatilla<br>Sepia |
| Fluid retention | decrease salt intake<br>diet<br>(rarely) diuretics<br>exercise<br>increase water intake | diet | dandelion<br>Dong Quai<br>green tea<br>nettle leaf<br>wild yam | Natrum mur |

Table 3. *Therapeutic Options in Perimenopause, Menopause, and Postmenopause (continued)*

| Problem | Medical | Complementary | Herbal | Homeopathic |
|---|---|---|---|---|
| Breast tenderness | diet<br>increase gamma<br>  linolenic acid<br>vitamin E | | black currant seed oil<br>black cohosh<br>borage oil<br>evening primrose<br>liferoot<br>vitex | Bryonia<br>Conium |
| Tricky gut | antispasmodic<br>bulking agents<br>charting<br>diet<br>exercise | | dandelion<br>fennel<br>fenugreek<br>ginger<br>psyllium<br>yellow dock root | Carbo vegetalis<br>Lycopodium<br>Nux vomica<br>Pulsatilla |

## MENOPAUSE

**Hot flashes, night sweats, and insomnia**

| diet | cold wipes | black cohosh | Belladonna |
|---|---|---|---|
| drugs | fans | chickweed | Coffea |
| HRT | layered natural fibers | dandelion | Ferrum metallicum |
| mineral supplements | separate beds | Dong Quai | Lachesis |
| | visualization | hops | Nux vomica |
| | | motherwort | Pulsatilla |
| | | oat straw | Sanguinaria |
| | | Ostaderm | Sepia |
| | | passion flower | Sulfur |
| | | raspberry | Sulfuricum acidicum |
| | | red clover | Valeriana |
| | | sage | |
| | | skullcap | |
| | | sweet flag bath | |
| | | valerian | |
| | | wild yam | |

Table 3. *Therapeutic Options in Perimenopause, Menopause, and Postmenopause* (continued)

| Problem | Medical | Complementary | Herbal | Homeopathic |
|---|---|---|---|---|
| Dryness | diet | | black cohosh | |
| | HRT | | calendula | |
| | lubricants: artificial | | comfrey | |
| | tears, saline spray | | cucumber slices on | |
| | | | eyes | |
| | oils | | Dong Quai | |
| | test for infection | | flax seed oil | |
| | | | motherwort | |
| | | | oat straw bath | |
| | | | Ostaderm V | |
| | | | tea bags on eyes | |
| | | | wild yam | |
| Decreased libido | ?DHEA | | Ostaderm | |
| | HRT | | | |
| | testosterone | | | |

| | | | | |
|---|---|---|---|---|
| Dizziness | breathe into cupped hands<br>diet<br>drugs<br>HRT | pacing yourself<br>taking time out<br>yoga | primula flower tea<br>smell lavender oil | Cocculus indicans |
| Formication<br>(see also Dryness) | anti-itch gels and creams<br>apply cold compresses | | dandelion<br>raw beets, grated or juice | Caladium<br>Rhus tox |
| Palpitations | drugs<br>mineral supplements<br>reassurance | relaxation | black haw<br>hawthorne<br>motherwort<br>valerian | Rock Rose<br>(Bach flower)<br>Spigelia |
| **POSTMENOPAUSE** | | | | |
| Dry vagina | lubricants with polycarbophil<br>Replens<br>topical estrogen<br>wild yam cream | massage daily with olive oil | comfrey ointment<br>Dong Quai<br>slippery elm<br>vaginal acidophilus capsules<br>wild yam cream | Belladonna<br>Bryonia<br>Lycopodium |

**Table 3.** *Therapeutic Options in Perimenopause, Menopause, and Postmenopause* (continued)

| Problem | Medical | Complementary | Herbal | Homeopathic |
|---|---|---|---|---|
| Burning, itchy vulvae and vagina | lubricants with polycarbophil<br>Replens<br>topical estrogen<br>wild yam cream | massage daily with olive oil | aloe vera gel<br>calendula cream<br>honey<br>motherwort<br>nettle tea<br>plantain ointment<br>wild yam cream | Belladonna<br>Cantharis<br>Natrum mur<br>Sulfur |
| Urethritis and cystitis | antibiotics<br>increase fluid intake<br>topical estrogen<br>urine culture and sensitivity test<br>vitamin C | cranberries and blueberries | echinacea<br>mallow<br>uva ursi<br>yarrow | Cantharis |

| | | | |
|---|---|---|---|
| Stress incontinence | biofeedback | black cohosh | Causticum |
| | diaphragm | catnip | Ferrum phos. |
| | diet | horsetail, agrimony, and sweet sumach combination | Pulsatilla |
| | double voiding | | |
| | HRT | | |
| | Kegel exercises | | |
| | physical therapy | | |
| | Reliance device | | |
| | scheduled toileting | | |
| | surgery | | |
| Hypertension | diet | dandelion | Crataegus |
| | drugs | garlic | Gelsemium |
| | exercise | hawthorne | Glonine |
| | HRT | motherwort | Natrum mur |
| | stop smoking | adequate calcium, magnesium, and potassium | Sulfur |
| | weight loss | meditation | |
| | | stress reduction techniques | |

**Table 3.** *Therapeutic Options in Perimenopause, Menopause, and Postmenopause* (continued)

| Problem | Medical | Complementary | Herbal | Homeopathic |
|---|---|---|---|---|
| Fractures and bone pain | calcium, magnesium, boron, and vitamin D | acupuncture | alfalfa | Arnica |
| | | home safety measures | comfrey poultices | Cuprum met. |
| | diet | tai chi | dandelion root | Nux vomica |
| | drugs | | horsetail | Rhus tox |
| | HRT | | kelp | Ruta |
| | TENS | | nettle | Silicea |
| | weight-bearing exercise | | oat straw | |
| | | | sage | |
| | | | skullcap | |
| | | | wild yam | |
| Foot and leg cramps | prescription quinine | calcium, magnesium, and vitamin E | black haw | Arsenicum |
| | | | oil of peppermint or rosemary bath | Chamomilla |
| | | tonic water | | Cuprum |
| | | | St. John's wort | Nux vomica |

| Wrinkles and droops | | |
| --- | --- | --- |
| avoid sun, smoking, alcohol | acceptance | nettle |
| diet | yoga | sage |
| chemical peels | | wild yam |
| face lifts | | |
| HRT | | |
| Renova cream | | |
| skin creams | | |
| sunscreen | | |

# CHAPTER 4

# Therapeutic Approaches in Perimenopause

## Menstrual Irregularity and PMS

Skipping months or bleeding every two weeks or bleeding heavily—any of these patterns can be considered menstrual irregularity, especially if this is a new pattern for you, a pattern different from the one you have grown used to in your adult years. You may have one or more of these irregular patterns during perimenopause. Although these patterns are both common and normal during perimenopause, any bleeding that is excessive or that occurs more frequently than your usual cycle should be checked out with your health care provider.

Charting your periods is an excellent way to identify your menstrual pattern. You can use the PMS chart that appears in Chapter 1. If you chart your periods for two or three months after noticing a change, you can then take your chart with you to your doctor's office, and he or she and you can go over it together. As a rule of thumb, changes that recur cyclically are usually normal. Also, if you can predict difficult days, you may be able to modify your life to accommodate them.

When periods become very heavy (called "flooding"), it's a good idea to rule out two common causes of excessive bleeding: iron deficiency and hypothyroidism. These imbalances can be diagnosed by common blood tests (serum iron, total iron-binding capacity, and ferritin tests, for iron deficiency, and a TSH test for levels of high-sensitivity thyroid-stimulating hormone, for hypothyroidism) and can be very easily treated with iron or thyroid hormone. If the results of these tests are normal, then there are three common possibilities: normal change of cycle due to fluctuating hormones in perimenopause; hyperplasia (a precancerous condition that must be monitored); and fibroid tumors.

There are many variations on common normal changes in cycle during perimenopause:

- change in the interval between periods (anywhere from three to six weeks is considered within normal range)
- change in the pattern of the flow, for example:
    initial spotting followed by one or two days of heavy flow
    a very brief period
    a much lighter period, either of normal length or shorter, followed by five to seven days of "chocolatey" spotting
- skipped periods

In addition to menstrual irregularities, a woman may develop PMS (premenstrual stress) for the first time, or she may begin having premenstrual symptoms again after not having had them for a while, or her premenstrual symptoms may get worse. Some women get cramps or acne, similar to the problems some adolescents have when their periods first begin.

## MEDICAL THERAPY FOR MENSTRUAL IRREGULARITY AND PMS

PMS vitamins, and specifically Optivite or Vita-PMS (which is a generic version of Optivite), have helped many women regulate their cycles in early perimenopause. And vitamin $B_6$ appears to help normalize the ratio of progesterone and estrogen in a woman's body: Guy Abraham, M.D., reported nearly thirty years ago that the administration of vitamin $B_6$ in doses of 200 to 800 mg daily can be helpful. You should only take high doses of $B_6$ (more than 300 mg) with the supervision of your health care provider, because this vitamin (like many others) can be toxic at high doses.

Magnesium levels may be low in women with PMS, and since magnesium deficiency has been shown to cause a depletion of brain dopamine, taking a magnesium supplement can be helpful (the PMS vitamins contain magnesium). Maintaining dopamine levels induces relaxation and increases mental alertness. Magnesium also eases premenstrual constipation and menstrual cramping. A regular exercise program (half an hour at least three times weekly) and a diet with only moderate amounts of sugar, salt, and caffeine also help, as does dividing your total daily calorie intake into six small feeds.

Ibuprofen, up to a maximum dose of 2400 mg daily, can be very helpful in stopping flooding. Ibuprofen has an antiprostaglandin effect, which helps control the bleeding. (Prostaglandins are hormone-like substances which may affect blood pressure, metabolism, and smooth muscle activity.) There are "good" and "bad" prostaglandins. In this case, the "good" prostaglandins help stimulate the contraction of the uterine muscle around the bleeding vessels, thereby shutting them off.

Menstrual symptoms can be controlled very well with combined estrogen/progesterone therapy or progesterone alone, or with oral contraceptives (which are a combination of estrogen and progesterone). But any woman with a pattern of excessive bleeding, and especially if the bleeding is not controlled by the simple measures described above, should not begin taking any hormonal therapy unless a transvaginal ultrasound or an endometrial biopsy or D&C have been performed. These procedures are performed to rule out endome-trial hyperplasia (a build up of the uterine lining), a condition that puts a woman at a significantly increased risk of develop-ing uterine cancer.

Sometimes a D&C, in which the lining of the uterus is scraped away, controls excessive bleeding for relatively long periods of time, and the procedure is commonly performed for this purpose; at the same time it allows the physician to check the womb for evidence of hyperplasia. A relatively re-cent option to control abnormal bleeding is endometrial abla-tion, a procedure in which the lining of the uterus is surgically stripped. This usually helps the bleeding but, according to a recent report, it is not a definitive cure for or protection against endometrial hyperplasia.

Fibroid tumors (often called simply fibroids) in the uterus are not uncommon at this stage of life. These tumors are not cancerous, but they may cause discomfort and may increase blood flow during periods or interrupt blood flow, depending upon how large they are and where they are located. Estrogens stimulate the fibroids to grow, so a woman who has fibroids and is taking hormone replacement therapy may have in-creased discomfort and bleeding. The role of estriol in fibroid growth is not clear, since estriol has both agonist and antago-nist activity: *agonist* in that it clearly has estrogenic effect in controlling symptoms and has positive effects on the cardio-vascular system, and *antagonist* in that studies show that it may protect the breast against the harmful effects of other estrogen (see Chapter 7). Certainly, for a woman with fibroid tumors, the wiser course is to avoid estrogens unless there are urgent reasons to use it, or unless the woman has decided to have a hysterectomy (surgery to remove the uterus) or myo-mectomy (surgery to remove the tumors).

## COMPLEMENTARY THERAPIES AND HERBS FOR MENSTRUAL IRREGULARITIES AND PMS

Acupuncture has been an extremely valuable part of my approach to both irregular menses and to flooding, especially when the flooding is due to fibroids. I have practiced acupuncture for about twenty years and have used it on a number of occasions to control bleeding in women who would otherwise have undergone a hysterectomy. It can also stimulate the onset of delayed menses and can be used to treat endometriosis. In acupuncture treatment, new, very fine needles are inserted in points in the body identified by centuries of practice as important for the specific bodily function being treated. It is a gentle, safe technique free of most side effects—though it does not always work.

Diet, as we have seen, is important for many aspects of menopause. Decreasing animal fat in the diet decreases an exogenous ("from outside") source of hormones, thereby avoiding stimulating the fibroids. (The animal hormones are thought to stimulate bleeding and discomfort.) Interestingly, most women tell me that they have lost interest in eating meat as they grow older. Fruits and vegetables can also expose you to estrogen-mimicking pesticides and herbicides, as can living in an agricultural area where a lot of spraying occurs. The best protection is eating organically grown produce and being aware of spraying practices in your community and advocating safety measures. We don't yet fully understand all the implications of exogenous sources of hormones such as diet and agricultural spraying, although links are being made between these agents and breast cancer and declining sperm counts.

*Phytosterols* are plant hormones. The human body can convert some phytosterols to human hormones, using the phytosterols as building material. Phytosterols can also be converted pharmacologically, to produce natural hormonal pharmaceuticals derived from soy and yams, for example.

The market is currently filled with a variety of forms and brand names of wild yam products. Table 4 lists a number of creams containing wild yam. I most commonly suggest the creams, but some of my patients prefer tinctures. My first exposure to these was about eight years ago, when Zena walked in with an article about Ostaderm, which she badly wanted to try but which was only sold through professional offices. I learned that Ostaderm was considered a cosmetic but was made by a naturopathic pharmacy. After reviewing the ingredients—which included aloe, licorice, soy, and wild yam—I ordered the cream for her, on a "won't hurt, might help" basis. She found it very helpful, in her case for headaches, residual hot flashes, and body aches.

Since that time, I have used wild yam creams with many of my patients. In early perimenopause, the wild yam/natural progesterone creams in the first group in Table 4 (creams containing more than 400 mg progesterone per ounce of cream) can be very helpful in regulating cycles and improving other symptoms. Apply 1/4 teaspoon twice daily to the face (it's also a good moisturizer), neck, belly, inner arms, or inner thighs. This provides a dose of phytoprogesterone (plant hormones that can be converted to progesterone) of about 35 mg, which smooths out the luteal phase of the menstrual cycle.

In women more advanced in their menopause, or when they slip out of control with the above creams, I suggest Ostaderm at a dose of 1/4 teaspoon twice every day. This cream gives the same approximate progesterone dose but also a small dose of phytoestrogen and, as far as I know, is the only cream that does this. Recently, George Roentsch, our local com-

**Table 4.** *Progesterone Content of Body Creams*

| Brand Name | Manufacturer | Progesterone (mg. per oz. of cream) | Location |
|---|---|---|---|
| CREAMS CONTAINING MORE THAN 400 MG. PROGESTERONE PER OZ. OF CREAM | | | |
| Alpine Progesterone | Jason Natural Cosmetics | 513 | Culver City, CA (310) 838-7543 |
| Angel Care | Angel Care USA | 658 | Atlanta, GA (770) 458-6111 |
| Angel Care | Angel Care USA | 640 | Atlanta, GA (770) 458-6111 |
| Angel Care | Angel Care USA | 644 | Atlanta, GA (770) 458-6111 |
| Balance Cream | Vitality Lifechoice | 517 | Carson City, NV (775) 882-6611 |
| Balance Cream | Vitality Lifechoice | 447 | Carson City, NV (775) 882-6611 |
| Balance Cream | Vitality Lifechoice | 470 | Carson City, NV (775) 882-6611 |
| DermaGest | Broadmoore Labs | 510 | Ventura, CA (800) 822-3712 |
| EssPro 7 | Young Living Essential | 463 | Payson, UT (800) 763-9963 |
| Femarone 17 | Wise Essentials | 536 | St. Paul, MN (800) 295-2256 |
| Fem-Gest | Bio-Nutritional Formulas | 431 | Mineola, NY (800) 950-8484 |
| Renascence Progesterone | Marpé International | 1586 | Johnson City, TN (800) 295-3477 |
| Maxine's Feminique | Country Life | 443 | Hauppauge, NY (800) 645-5768 |
| NatraGest | Broadmoore Labs | 446 | Ventura, CA (800) 822-3712 |
| Ostaderm | Bezwecken | 400 | Beaverton, OR (503) 644-7800 |

# Table 4. *Progesterone Content of Body Creams* (continued)

| Brand Name | Manufacturer | Progesterone (mg. per oz. of cream) | Location |
|---|---|---|---|
| Procreme | THG Health Products | 489 | Oxford, PA (800) 677-7694 |
| Procreme Plus | THG Health Products | 926 | Oxford, PA (800) 677-7694 |
| Progest | Bezwecken | 400 | Beaverton, OR (503) 644-7800 |
| Progesterone Cream | Jason Natural Cosmetics | 496 | Culver City, CA (301) 838-7543 |
| Progesterone Max | Jason Natural Cosmetics | 402 | Culver City, CA (301) 838-7543 |
| ProL'eve | Brain Garden | 542 | Provo, UT (800) 481-9987 |
| SupraGest | Health Alternatives West | 452 | Ventura, CA (877) 984-9286 |
| Wild Yam Crème with Progesterone | Wise Woman Essentials | 525 | St. Paul, MN (800) 295-2256 |

CREAMS CONTAINING LESS THAN 400 MG. PROGESTERONE PER OZ. OF CREAM

| | | | |
|---|---|---|---|
| Progesterone Cream | Jason Natural Products | 274 | Culver City, CA (800) 838-7543 |

CREAMS CONTAINING 5 MG. OR LESS PROGESTERONE PER OZ. OF CREAM

| | | | |
|---|---|---|---|
| Femarone | Wise Essentials | None | St. Paul, MN (800) 295-2256 |
| Ultra Harmony | Wise Woman Essentials | 0.85 | St. Paul, MN (800) 295-2256 |

*Note:* The creams were tested by an independent HPLC laboratory and confirmed by RIA at Aeron. Manufacturers pay an annual membership fee for administrative costs of the PIC program as well as a testing fee for each batch of new product. Aeron certifies that the cream products listed above contain the stated amount of progesterone. Aeron assumes no responsibility for the performance of the products tested. This listing is produced as a service to consumers interested in knowing the progesterone content in topical creams and lotions. *Source:* Aeron Life Cycles Clinical Laboratory, June 15, 1999. Reproduced by permission.

pounding pharmacist, made up a cream containing black cohosh and natural progesterone. This provides an intermediate dose between the over-the-counter creams and prescription-strength creams.

Both over-the-counter creams and prescription-strength creams have been very effective in regulating cycles when appropriately selected. Ostaderm may stimulate fibroids, but this is unusual.

Herbs that contain phytoestrogens (plant hormones that can be converted to estrogen) are Dong Quai, raspberry leaf (rose family), black cohosh, hops, licorice root, pomegranate seeds, and sage. Herbs high in phytoprogesterones (plant hormones that can be converted to progesterone) are vitex (chaste tree berry), wild yam roots, yarrow, and sarsaparilla. Having a greater understanding of which herbs are likely to improve which conditions helps us make good choices among various herbal remedies (see below for more information about specific herbal remedies).

Herbal estrogenic sources have estrogen-like properties but do not pose the risks of estrogen; they are also not as potent as estrogen. Herbal estrogenic sources often help to regulate the cycle and decrease spotting. The herbal estrogenic sources are Dong Quai, wheat germ oil, and raspberry leaf.

Dong Quai is often listed in herb books or field guides as *Angelica sinensis*. A member of the parsley family, it has long been used in Asian medicine. One or more close relatives of Dong Quai may be growing in your garden or field. While they make reasonable substitutes, you need to be sure that you have properly identified the plant before eating it.

Dong Quai is strongly estrogenic. It has been very effective for many women in regulating menopausal symptoms, and its effectiveness has recently been verified in herbal clinical research. It can be used in a variety of ways:

- ½ to 1 cup of tea
- up to 40 drops of tincture
- ¼ inch of dried root, chewed like gum
- capsules (follow the dosage on the bottle)

Wheat germ oil is a good source of vitamin E, which common wisdom has held to be estrogenic and helpful for a wide variety of menopausal woes. Recent studies have not validated this notion about the effectiveness of vitamin E, however—there was no statistical difference between vitamin E and placebo (sugar pill). But what's wrong with the placebo effect?

Wheat germ is a food and can be liberally ingested. It is a good source not just of vitamin E but also of the "good" fats and fiber.

Raspberry leaf, along with other members of the rose family, is rich in *bioflavonoids*. Bioflavonoids are a class of chemical found in nature which has measurable estrogenic activity as well as antioxidant, anti-inflammatory, and antihistaminic effects. Bioflavonoids are also necessary to the health and strength of the capillaries and to the utilization of vitamin C. They make very pleasant teas.

Cinnamon is a very useful remedy for cycles plagued by spotting or flooding. When these are a problem, I suggest women make cinnamon tea, steep cinnamon in any warm beverage that they enjoy, and use powdered cinnamon—lots of it—on just about anything. Cinnamon flavoring or potpourri oils should not be used because these are often synthetic and may be toxic. Cinnamon is a very pleasant remedy but, like anything spicy, may aggravate hot flashes in some women. Although I don't know how or why it works pharmacologically, I have often observed that it does. This bit of wisdom was passed to me by my grandmother, Rosealba Keib.

Gamma linolenic acid (GLA) is found in evening primrose

oil, black currant seed oil, and borage oil, and is necessary for your body to make anti-inflammatory prostaglandins. (As mentioned above, ibuprofen also acts on the prostaglandins.) Gamma linolenic acid can be helpful, because of this action, as a therapeutic for excessive bleeding and for breast tenderness. Flax seed is rich in GLA and the Omega 3 fatty acids (one of the "good" fats), as well. I suggest to most of my patients that they grind two tablespoons of flax seed daily and sprinkle it over yogurt, salads, cereals, and so on. It is the cheapest and most palatable way to ingest GLA. I also bake the ground flax seed, or meal, into my breads, as has been done in Europe for generations. It also gives you a "good coat"—shiny hair, moisture-replete skin, and a healthy glow.

The combination I most commonly suggest for women with fibroids and flooding due to fibroids is vitex tincture (forty drops total per day), cinnamon, and visualization. Vitex (chaste tree berry) has been used for women's menstrual disorders for many centuries, and recent research, published mostly in German journals, has verified its usefulness in luteal phase disorders, including menorrhagia (abnormally heavy menstrual flow) due to fibroids or to progesterone deficiency. Vitex also slowly smooths out many other menopausal symptoms. Cinnamon used together with vitex helps stop flooding more quickly. Try sucking on a cinnamon stick all day!

To practice visualization, get comfortable in a quiet place and focus your thoughts. Or focus your thoughts while sitting in a doctor's waiting room—or any place. I personally don't like using negative images for visualization, so I don't suggest using any images of violence being done to your fibroids. Instead, I like images of flowers coming to fruition and then, quite naturally, dropping from their stalks. Or any image that is particularly meaningful for you.

Shepherd's-purse and lady's mantle are truly fast-acting

remedies for flooding. A recent study on several hundred women showed that lady's mantle controlled hemorrhage, with a peak effect within three to five days. Shepard's purse acts even more quickly, by causing the uterus to contract down and, basically, clamp the bleeding vessels closed. It is taken as tea, and results are seen within a few hours to two days.

Witch hazel is also good for acute flooding and can be used as a tincture. It acts a little differently, by increasing tone in the uterine muscles.

Yellow dock root and dandelion are excellent sources of iron. As previously discussed, low iron levels can trigger excessive bleeding, so every woman should make sure she gets enough iron. Both yellow dock root and dandelion also contain vitamin C, which you need to utilize iron, calcium, and magnesium in your body. Dandelion leaves can be eaten— young and tender in salads, or steamed and served as a warm green. They can also be prepared as a tea. Yellow dock root is most often used as a tincture.

## HOMEOPATHIC THERAPIES FOR MENSTRUAL IRREGULARITIES

Belladonna is used for profuse bleeding of bright red blood, painful cramps, and perhaps offensive odor.

China is for painless blackish hemorrhage.

Crocus sativa is for painless, profuse, blackish bleeding with clots and offensive odor. Body feels cold.

Ipecacuanha is for bright red continuous flooding. Symptoms may also include cramps, vomiting, and general weakness.

Lachesis is the most beneficial remedy for excessive flow. Commonly associated symptoms treated by lachesis are headache, flushing, fatigue, chest tightness, and cold hands and feet.

Natrum mur (sea salt) is for irregular, prolonged periods,

cramps, constipation, and headaches, and for flooding associated with depression and exhaustion.

Secale is for flooding without clots but with bad cramping.

Sepia is useful in treating late periods that are either very
heavy or scanty and that are associated with backache and
bearing-down pain, feeling like the pelvic organs will fall out.
The symptoms feel better at midday and afternoon and are
improved by very hard exercise. Irritability and depression are
also helped by sepia.

Sulfur is for flooding, hot flashes, and sweats.

If these measures do not help and you are soaking through a
pad or tampon in less than an hour, you should see your
health care practitioner or an urgent care center as soon as
possible. Heavy bleeding may be life-threatening. Don't delay.

Another thing to keep in mind is that, although fertility
declines as we reach our forties, we must still consider ourselves fertile and use appropriate contraception if we wish to
avoid a surprise pregnancy. Recently, a forty-five-year-old patient of mine had scheduled a visit to discuss having tubal
ligation surgery, only to have an initial prenatal visit, instead!

## Aches and Pains

Nobody likes to ache. It makes us feel tired, grumpy, old,
and fearful. An important preventive is to learn to honor our
body's own rhythm of activity and quiet that allows for work
and rest. Easy to say, harder to do. Too often we mind only the
"to do" agenda and its time constraints.

Exercise, too, is very helpful in preventing and decreasing
joint and muscle achiness. Ideally, you'll get both aerobic and
stretching types of exercise. Walking and yoga are a good combination. Modern dance is great because it contains elements

of both aerobic and stretching exercises. To release all your creative energy, you might try African dancing or belly dancing. Both are lots of fun. In fact, fun should be part of your exercise routine.

A "lube job" for stiff bodies is always a good idea. In this case it means making sure that you're getting Omega 3 and Omega 6 fatty acids, two of the "good" fats. These fatty acids supply the precursors for our bodies to make anti-inflammatory prostaglandins. A diet high in fatty fish (salmon, tuna, mackerel, bluefish, herring, sardines) and fresh seeds, nuts, and grains and vegetables with canola oil can provide these fatty acids. Or you can supplement with two tablespoons of ground flax seeds and one borage oil capsule every day. If your muscles are aching or cramping (do you get a charley horse at night? or cramping feet?), you may need to supplement with calcium, magnesium, and vitamin E. These also help the restless legs that can disturb your sleep. Usually, 1,000 mg calcium, 500 mg magnesium, and 600 IU of vitamin E do the trick.

Regularly scheduled massage, acupuncture, or therapeutic touch are very pleasant ways of dealing with this "minor malady of menopause." All of them, in addition to be being therapeutic, increase your sense of well-being and provide deep relaxation. Acupuncture has been shown to raise endorphin levels and can be effective for severe and chronic pain. If you've never had a massage, do! It gets the kinks out of the muscles while bringing back memories of your mother rubbing your back, or conjuring up the feeling of the warmth of sun or the slide of water on your skin in a bath. A facial is another wonderful way to relieve tension. Any form of deep heat feels great; moxibustion is one that many acupuncturists use. "Moxa" is like incense and is burned over the acupuncture points.

If absolutely necessary, one can use drugs to relieve aches

and pains. Over-the-counter drugs usually do the trick. The salicylates, including aspirin, enteric-coated aspirin, topical rubs like Ben-Gay, and willow bark teas can all be effective. So, too, can the nonaspirin, nonsteroidal anti-inflammatory drugs (NSAIDs) like ibuprofen, naproxen, and ketoprofen. All of them relieve inflammation (swelling, redness, and heat) as well as pain. Acetaminophen products (such as Tylenol) relieve pain but do not relieve inflammation. Judicious use of any of these may be helpful, but if you find yourself relying on them to get through a day, you should see your doctor and set up a more effective program for pain relief.

Homeopathic remedies that may be helpful are Arnica and Rhus tox. Arnica is good for muscle aches and is available as a topical cream as well as in oral preparations. Rhus tox is better for the joint aches and may be quite helpful.

Dong Quai, as well as other phytoestrogen donors, may be helpful for minor joint aches. St. John's wort can help by relaxing achy muscles and increasing available serotonin. Kava-Kava may also promote muscle relaxation.

## Migraines

Migraine headaches, to me, are a foretaste of hell. My acquaintance with this scourge began in my early forties and escalated until menopause. We all can characterize these headaches as different from other, more minor ones. Mine was always the ice pick in the right eye. Needless to say, I became very interested in ways to avoid and treat migraines.

### MEDICAL THERAPY FOR MIGRAINES

The first step in solving a problem is to define it. For migraines, this involves menstrual charting (use the PMS chart in Chapter 1) and keeping a daily diary in which you note the foods you ate, the drinks you drank, the events you attended or participated in, and the emotions you experienced. Charting allows you to see connections between your hormonal cycles and your migraines, and your diary hints of connections between the pattern of migraines and what you ingest, do, and feel.

I was really quite typical of many women. I would get a migraine two or three days before my period and it would last, in varying intensity, until flow began. Some women also have a routine migraine at ovulation. Other triggers for me—and for many other women—were any form of alcoholic beverage (no matter the quantity), not eating enough, too long an interval between meals, too little fluid intake during the day, the combination of sweets and coffee, coffee by itself in excess of one cup of regular coffee, and physical stressors, such as too much sun ( I now always wear sunglasses while driving) or too much heat. Some women are very sensitive to emotional triggers, but emotions rarely triggered my headaches, although fatigue would. Odors, such as cigarette smoke, perfumes, paint, and glue, could lay me out for several days. The classical food triggers for migraine are foods high in tyramine, for example, beer, aged cheese, banana, chocolate, red wine, soy sauce, and dried fish. Oranges and tomato may also be triggers.

Once you have kept your chart and your diary for a couple of months, you are ready to begin preventive measures. But first take a critical look at your self-expectations. Most of us assume that we should be fully "on" all the time, and that we don't need to pay any attention to physiologic cycling. We have heard our cycles used as reason for not trusting women in high office or as CEO or whatever position we might aspire to. We can meet our obligations and still honor our rhythms, however. An honest look at these obligations will reveal that a core of chores are necessary each day, but that while the rest of the items on our "to do" list may *feel* pressing, they can really be spread out over other days.

Be a wee bit neglectful of nonessential chores on your delicate days. Feel no guilt; remember that the migraine will force you to be even more neglectful and may even make you non-functional. Enlist the cooperation of family and friends and co-workers, and be respectful of their "delicate days" in return (we all have them—men, too). Be sure, on your delicate days, to get extra rest, miss no meals, and avoid your particular triggers. This would be a great time for a massage or therapeutic touch.

Obviously, as a physician, I have seen many women trying to deal with migraines. Rarely do I prescribe any drugs for this problem beyond ibuprofen, aspirin, or the occasional Fiorinal-type drug, because other measures can, and do, work. With very few exceptions, acupuncture has helped as both treatment and prevention in those of my patients who choose this approach. Usually, I treat patients with acupuncture at weekly intervals for three to four weeks, and then in the week prior to each cycle, as needed. We generally find that after the first two or three months, three or four visits each year continues to prevent migraine. This is true for acupuncture for menstrual cramping, as well.

For a number of women, I have found that addressing the hormonal connection can make a huge difference. In the peri-menopausal phase, I'll often suggest a trial of Ostaderm cream, usually one-quarter teaspoon twice daily. This is often at least partially effective. At other times, the patient and I may opt for hormone replacement. I always have transdermal (patch), gel, or cream progesterone compounded for women with migraine, because experience has taught me that most women get more frequent or more severe migraines when taking oral progestins, but usually they can tolerate a transdermal. Oral estriol and estradiol seem less likely to cause migraine than other forms of estrogen.

## HERBAL AND HOMEOPATHIC APPROACHES TO RELIEVING AND PREVENTING MIGRAINE

Herbal remedies for migraine include feverfew, black cohosh, skullcap, and St. John's wort. Much has been written lately about the usefulness of feverfew in treating migraine, and indeed, studies of its effectiveness in migraine are currently being done. It is emerging that feverfew is effective for the treatment of migraine, specifically in decreasing the frequency and severity of the attacks. Two or three fresh leaves chewed daily, or one capsule, standardized at 0.25 to 0.5 mg daily, have been shown to be effective in preventing migraine; much higher doses are needed to relieve pain in an acute attack.

Sage and black cohosh are both sources of phytoestrogen and, as such, may be effective for hormone-related migraines. I would lean toward a combination of black cohosh and wild yam cream or tincture, providing both phytoestrogen and phytoprogestin and thereby acting similarly to hormone replacement.

Skullcap and St. John's wort both have sedative, antispasmodic, and anti-inflammatory properties and may be very helpful during a migraine. One to three teaspoons of the tincture is likely to be more effective for relief of headache than making an infusion or tea. Willow is an excellent source of salicylates (aspirin-like compounds). Willow leaf vinegar or willow bark infusion can be used.

Homeopathic remedies for migraine include Lycopodium, Natrum mur, and Pulsatilla, as well as Spigelia and others.

Lycopodium is a homeopathic remedy that may help a right-sided migraine, especially occurring in late afternoon or early evening and triggered by missing a meal. Natrum mur (sea salt) may help the throbbing, vise-like headache, worse in the morning and with movement. Pulsatilla is used for a right-sided headache starting at the top of the head and associated with being too warm. The headache may be accompanied by tearing, especially of the right eye.

Sanguinaria helps the right-sided headache, beginning at the base of the skull and neck and settling in the right eye area. This headache may be associated with a stomachache and is aggravated by the sun or light. It gets better after vomiting and sleeping. Silica may help the migraine aggravated by alcohol, noise, and excitement. This headache may be associated with vertigo and blurred vision. Spigelia is for a left-sided headache associated with pain around the left eye, heart palpitations, and dizziness. Thuja is also useful for a left-sided headache, sharp at the back of the skull. (Thujone is one of the active properties in sage.)

## Problem with Short-Term Memory

When I was in medical school, I used to keep my life in order in a simple little Hallmark datebook. For many years, the calendar at home and my secretary at work had replaced this datebook system. Then I found myself in the store, at age forty-nine, buying a brain! Mine was not electronic, although the electronic "brains" are nice. Mine was a three-inch by six-inch leatherette diary that fit in my purse. In this I duly recorded all dates, obligations, important lists, and so on. You, too, can save your sanity and image with this low-tech device.

If your life doesn't already entail activities in which you do a lot of word recall, it is also important to keep your mind engaged with such things as crossword puzzles, singing, or reciting poetry. Memory exercises are described in several popular books written to help people improve their memory.

Estrogen sources can be very helpful to the memory. Hormone replacement therapy, Dong Quai, black cohosh, and Ostaderm cream can be considered. A homeopathic remedy is Lycopodium.

Gingko biloba has been shown to increase cerebral blood flow and to improve cognitive functions. The minimum dose is 120 mg daily; the dose that has been studied more closely is 240 mg daily.

## Emotional Turmoil

As I mentioned earlier, a circle of women friends is the single most therapeutic intervention during the menopausal years. This can range from a lunch-time grouping of friends at work to a formal support group. It is fun, unifying, and uplifting to sing with a group, to dance—Mediterranean, African, circle dancing—and to open yourself to joy. Run barefoot through wet grass. Lie flat and smell the earth. Start seedlings in midwinter. Play a musical instrument. Swim!

Undoubtedly, your family has noticed that you are a wee bit volatile. Enlist their understanding by explaining what's happening for you and sharing educational materials with them. Your partner may be very relieved to know that any libido changes are not a personal reflection on him or her. If you find that you are less orgasmic now and that this bothers your partner much more than it does you, he or she may need to hear that in the presence of a third party. I have seen this work in my practice.

Quiet time to yourself is essential now. Think of it as gestating time for the changes that are happening in you and as meditative time to guide these changes. Pursue your creative interests. Have a massage or facial. Keep a journal.

Seek a rhythm to your life and activities. Notice your breathing: you can not inhale without exhaling, and vice versa. Ideally, your life should be like this, too—a balance of activities and rest, function and creativity, external and internal. Exercise can be very beneficial to mood.

For some women, the intensity of this time, as well as the life events they bring to it, makes counseling necessary and extremely beneficial. Women do best working with women therapists at this stage of life, and tremendous personal growth can be achieved. Rarely, a woman may require pharmaceutical intervention, possibly including antidepressants, above and beyond addressing the hormones.

Androgens such as DHEA and testosterone are often helpful in alleviating depression in menopausal women for whom estrogen has not been sufficient. These should be monitored by blood levels and, if natural testosterone is used, one must remain mindful that this converts at a variable rate to estradiol, and that estradiol must also be monitored.

For herbal therapy to treat depression, consider the plants containing phytoestrogens, such as motherwort, black cohosh, and sage, and plants containing phytoprogestins, such as wild yam and vitex. Wild yam and vitex are obviously specific to the hormonal triggers, and these are often remedy enough.

Valerian, passion flower, and motherwort can be soothing and calming. Kava-Kava is used as a ceremonial drink in the South Pacific and produces a very mellow state of mind without impairing reasoning or function. It should not be used habitually, however, because it may damage the liver. St. John's wort is very useful for depression. Studies have shown it to be as effective as the selective serotonin reuptake inhibitor drugs (such as Prozac) in mild to moderate depression, and with fewer side effects.

Ginseng is an adaptogen and mimics or stimulates adrenal activity. It can be a powerful mood elevator, but it can also raise blood pressure. Most of the commercially available teas are quite safe in normal usage.

Homeopathic remedies for depression include Aurum met, which is indicated for depression with hopelessness and extreme irritability and when the symptoms are worse during the night, possibly with night sweats and palpitations. Calcarea is for depression and excessive worry about health. Caulophyllum is for nervous tension and anxiety. Cimifuga is for a gloomy, nervous, excitable mood. Natrum mur (sea salt) is for weepy and withdrawn, possibly with vertigo. Phosphorus is for excitable and easily irritated, with vertigo and chest tightness.

Pulsatilla is for lack of assertiveness or self-confidence, discouragement, whininess, and Sepia is for irritabilty, sulkiness, oversensitivity, anxiety. Calms forte is a proprietary mixture for anxiety and insomnia. (A proprietary mixture is a trademarked mixture of several homeopathic remedies.)

## Fluid Retention

The three foundations for combating fluid retention are (1) a healthy diet (one that is low in salt and sugar and does not contain excessive calories); (2) adequate exercise; and (3) adequate water intake, which means drinking eight to ten eight-ounce glasses daily. *Be sure you drink eight to ten eight-ounce glasses every day.* Keeping your body well hydrated means your body won't try to "hold on" to fluid in response to detecting low amounts of fluid in the system. The next step is to add two to three cups of green tea daily. Green tea is an antioxidant source and a natural diuretic (as are oolong and black tea). These approaches are so effective that I very seldom prescribe a diuretic.

Asparagus, lettuce, grapes, cucumber, watermelon, and cantaloupe are foods that have high water content, high fiber content, and low sodium content, and so help to reduce fluid retention in the tissues. Herbal helpers are dandelion tea or tincture, nettle leaf infusion, Dong Quai, and wild yam tincture or cream. Natrum mur (sea salt) may be useful as a homeopathic remedy.

## Breast Tenderness

Breast tenderness is a common complaint throughout our menstrual lives, as well as in menopausal years. In my experience, this symptom usually responds dramatically to a decreased caffeine and salt intake and an increased intake of gamma linolenic acid. The least expensive way to get more gamma linolenic acid in your diet is to use canola oil, flax seed oil (one tablespoon daily), or ground flax seeds (two tablespoons daily). If these don't work for you or if you choose not to use them, then borage oil capsules (one or two daily), evening primrose oil capsules (three to six daily), or black currant seed oil capsules (three to six daily) will usually provide relief.

I have not had the need to suggest remedies other than these, but, in the herbal tradition, black cohosh, vitex, and liferoot have a reputation for being helpful, and Conium and Bryonia are homeopathic aids.

## Tricky Gut

Tricky gut is my term for the maddening and sometimes debilitating digestive symptoms many women experience at this time in their lives. There may have been hints about what's to come: the common complaint of constipation in the week preceding menses and, equally common, the frequent urination at the onset of bleeding, accompanied by loose stools or a little diarrhea.

It is apparent that some women begin to have digestive difficulties in their forties and fifties. Symptoms can range from heartburn to diarrhea, with many shades in between. For some, the symptoms warrant a medical work-up to rule out serious pathology; for others, it may be a matter of "I obviously can't eat onions (or beans, or whatever) anymore." Most women who come to see me with these symptoms have been diagnosed as having irritable bowel syndrome and are looking for a helpful diet.

For a woman who does not have any disease to account for digestive difficulties, a four-day rotation diet, coupled with a diet diary, is a useful tool in dealing with a tricky gut. Following the diet for two to three weeks, while charting symptoms and foods eaten each day, allows us to pick up hints of foods or food families that may be troublesome—and then avoid them. If dairy foods are the problem, try adding lactase to milk and other dairy products before eating them. (It is not uncommon to lose tolerance for lactose at this stage in life.) Likewise, the product called Beano sometimes helps in digesting beans. The four-day rotation diet presented in Table 5 was created by Esther Breckenridge, R.N., my office nurse.

It is almost too obvious to state that plenty of water, exercise, and a decent diet are basic requirements. If your diet is coffee and cigs for breakfast, diet soda for lunch, and fast food

**Table 5.** *Four-Day Rotation Diet*

Follow this diet for two or three weeks. After day 4, begin again with day 1, and so on. Keep a record of what you eat and try to identify which food or category of food gives you a problem.

Eat as much as you want of the foods in each category each day, but eat only from the choices listed in each category for that day. If you eat pork on day 1, for example, you will not get a clear idea of what's causing your problem.

Keep in mind that this diet is designed solely for the purpose of identifying troublesome foods. It is not a diet designed for healthy eating (coconut oil, for example, is very high in saturated fat, so you may want to avoid it altogether). If you are on a prescribed diet for health reasons, you will want to check with your doctor before starting any new diet.

|  | *Day 1* | *Day 2* | *Day 3* | *Day 4* |
|---|---|---|---|---|
| Protein | beef | bluefish | chicken | shellfish |
|  | lamb | mackerel | duck | whitefish |
|  | rabbit | pork | eggs |  |
|  | veal | salmon | game hen |  |
|  |  | tuna | turkey |  |
| Fruits | apricot | coconut | banana | apple |
|  | avocado | date | blackberry | blueberry |
|  | cherry | grape | loganberry | cranberry |
|  | fig | kiwi | raspberry | currant |
|  | peach | persimmon | strawberry | pear |
|  | plum | pineapple |  | quince |
|  | prune | pomegranate |  |  |
|  | rhubarb | raisin |  |  |
| Oils | apricot | coconut | sunflower | flax |
|  | butter | olive | walnut | sesame |
|  | canola (rape) | safflower |  | soy |
| Vegetables | asparagus | artichoke | bok choy | beans (all) |
|  | eggplant | carrot | broccoli | beet |

**Table 5.** *Four-Day Rotation Diet* (continued)

|  | Day 1 | Day 2 | Day 3 | Day 4 |
|---|---|---|---|---|
|  | garlic | celery | Brussel sprouts | peas (all) |
|  | okra | cucumber | cabbage | spinach |
|  | onion | dandelion | cauliflower | Swiss chard |
|  | potato | lettuce | collard greens |  |
|  | peppers (all) | parsley | plantain |  |
|  | tomato | parsnip | radish |  |
|  |  | pumpkin | turnip |  |
|  |  | squash |  |  |
| Seeds and nuts | almond | cashew | dulse | chestnut |
|  | Brazil nut | pistachio | pecans | filbert |
|  | macadamia | pumpkin seed | sunflower seed | hazelnut |
|  |  | vanilla | walnut | sesame seed |
| Spice and herbs | allspice | caraway | basil | lemon |
|  | bay leaf | coriander | cardamom | lime |
|  | chives | dill | ginger | mace |
|  | cinnamon | parsley | marjoram | nutmeg |
|  | clove | tarragon | mint | orange |
|  | paprika |  | mustard |  |
|  |  |  | oregano |  |
|  |  |  | rosemary |  |
|  |  |  | sage |  |
|  |  |  | savory |  |
|  |  |  | thyme |  |
| Starch or grain | buckwheat | bamboo shoot | agar-agar | arrowroot |
|  | potato flour | barley | amaranth | quinoa |
|  | spelt |  | cream of tartar | sesame meat |
|  |  |  |  | soy |

Table 5.  *Four-Day Rotation Diet* (continued)

| Day 1 | Day 2 | Day 3 | Day 4 |
|-------|-------|-------|-------|
| | millet | Jerusalem | |
| | oat | artichoke | |
| | rice | kamut (an | |
| | rye | ancient | |
| | wheat | grain, now | |
| | | available | |
| | | again) | |
| | | sweet potato | |
| | | tapioca | |
| | | teff | |
| | | water | |
| | | chestnut | |

for dinner, then you know yourself that a return to basics is called for.

Patterns of eating also contribute to distress. Most of us would feel best eating a small amount every two to three hours. To maintain a steady blood sugar level, combine some complex carbohydrate with a small amount of fat or protein. For example, an apple quarter with a thin skim of nut butter or low fat cream cheese. Or, a decadent favorite of mine, a cooked prune stuffed with a little bit of peanut butter. Light meals and adequate snacks help a lot. *Don't neglect breakfast.*

Bulking agents such as psyllium, methyl cellulose, ground flax seeds, oat bran, and pectin can be helpful for women who have problems with constipation and diarrhea. They are worth trying, even if you think that you already eat a "rabbit" diet consisting of nothing but bulk and fiber. Magnesium can be a helpful adjunct, too, but it will trigger diarrhea if the dose is excessive; 300 mg to 500 mg usually suffices.

Trial and error sometimes demonstrates the helpfulness of digestive enzymes such as lactase and Beano. Once in a while I prescribe an antispasmodic such as dicyclomine, to settle the bowel.

Many women are amazed to find that these symptoms markedly decrease or even vanish when they begin hormonal therapy.

Herbal approaches to the gut problem are similar to the measures already discussed. Ginger can be very helpful for nausea, vague stomach discomfort, and feelings of acidity. Most of us were offered ginger ale as children, so why not now? I more often will pour boiling water over a slice of fresh or crystallized ginger and let it steep a bit. Or one can buy ginger tea bags.

Yellow dock root tincture or dandelion leaves or root tincture can be very effective for gas or constipation. What could be more pleasant in early spring than a salad of early sorrel and tender young dandelion greens! Add a little balsamic vinegar and olive oil, a few johnny jump-ups, and no gourmet has feasted better.

Chewing fennel or fenugreek seeds helps relieve the embarrassment of gas. You may still have some gas but it will not have an offensive odor.

Homeopathic remedies for tricky gut include Carbo vegetalis, which is useful for acid indigestion accompanied by nausea, flatulence, and tummy ache when these symptoms are triggered by food. Lycopodium is indicated for flatulence associated with noisy rumblings, nausea, and sudden need to eat immediately. Any delay leads to a drained and empty sensation.

Nux vomica is useful in chronic constipation in which laxatives have been abused. This condition is often accompanied by nausea and irritability. There is a heavy, full feeling, worse in the morning, often associated with heavy eating and little exercise. Pulsatilla is helpful when you crave carbohydrates and then feel dry, when the food feels stuck in the middle of your chest, and when you also feel bloated and puffy.

Among these many remedies, I hope you will find relief of your own symptoms.

# CHAPTER 5

# Therapeutic Approaches in Menopause

Many of the therapeutic approaches to symptoms of peri-menopause were covered in the previous chapter. This chapter covers symptoms that occur mainly in menopause. (You can refer to Table 3, which is a complete list of symptoms and therapeutics throughout perimenopause, menopause, and postmenopause.)

## Hot Flashes, Night Sweats, and Insomnia

I have great sympathy for every woman lying awake at night. During the day, it is easier to appreciate a hot flash as a "power surge" and to affirm your status as a new woman, but somehow resources wane in the depths of night.

Small practical things help many women: changing from synthetic fibers to all-cotton nighties, keeping a fan blowing obliquely on your side of the bed, keeping wipes or a cool, damp washcloth handy, and dividing your bedding or using separate beds. Visualization can truly help; my personal favorites were a waterfall, floating in a river, sliding on snow, and standing in a breeze.

For most of the hormonal symptoms, hormone replacement will, of course, be helpful.

Pharmaceutically, Bellergal and Clonidine have been used to help with hot flashes. Bellergal is a drug that acts non-specifically on the autonomic (or involuntary) nervous system. Because it contains phenobarbital, some fear its addictive potential. I've never encountered this in my patients, however. Clonidine is an antihypertensive drug that decreases the peripheral resistance in the vascular system, which probably explains how it helps with hot flashes. I have not prescribed this drug as a treatment for hot flashes. The class of drugs known as selective serotonin reuptake inhibitors (SSRIS), including Prozac, Paxil, and Celexa, are used by many doctors to treat the symptoms of menopause. These are antidepressants and may help with some symptoms, but like many other drugs, they are not as effective as hormones. Also, for the woman who is taking Tamoxifen for breast cancer, this class of drug may not be a good choice because they interfere with effective blood levels of Tamoxifen.

For sleep disturbance not associated with night sweats or hot flashes, a nighttime dose of magnesium or a calcium/magnesium dose is often helpful. Melatonin may be helpful at doses of 1.5 to 3 mg. Five-hydroxytryptophan is available by prescription and can be very helpful in a bedtime dose of 50 mg. I am a bit wary of the over-the-counter versions of metabolites, because recently a contaminant was identified in some. It is rare that I prescribe hypnotics, and usually before doing so I will suggest a trial of Benadryl, since this makes many women sleepy.

Herbal remedies include bathing in a tepid or warm bath that has been scented with sweet flag, especially in the middle of the night. Try aromatherapy with basil or thyme oils (this never worked for me, but to each her own).

Again, it is the phytoestrogen-donating herbs that are most helpful. Black cohosh, motherwort, Dong Quai, and mixes of red clover and raspberry lead the pack, but oat straw, dandelion, and chickweed are also helpful. My patients have gotten relief by using Ostaderm, which contains aloe, licorice, soy, and wild yam. Sage contains thujones, which decrease sweating. Try a cup of sage tea at night. Prepare it by boiling one teaspoon of sage with two cups of water.

For insomnia, valerian alone or in combination with hops, skullcap, or passion flower can be helpful, taken about half an hour before bedtime. It is also very important to clear the last hour of your day from all " busyness" and to have a routine or bedtime ritual, much as we do with young children.

Homeopathic aids include Belladonna, Pulsatilla, and Sulfur, plus many more. Belladonna is for the red faced, jerking out of a heavy sleep, nightmares, hot sweats. Coffea is for mind racing, awaken at any sound, overstimulated. Ferrum metallicum for confused, vivid dreams, for restless sleep, difficulty falling asleep.

Lachesis is for hot flashes when falling asleep and awakening, sweaty during sleep, flushes of heat. Nux vomica for red, turgid face; sleeplessness with overabundance of ideas; awakens early and can't return to sleep; awakens unrefreshed; nightmares. Pulsatilla for frequent need to urinate at night, discomfort lying down, awakens unrefreshed. Sanguinaria for burning heat; red, hot cheeks; flushes of heat into head and face; with headache, little sweat. Sepia for sweating easily or for weakness followed by anxiety and hot flashes.

Sulfur is for hot flashes; sweating in armpits and on hands and feet; itchiness, especially at night; hot feet; unrefreshing sleep. Sulphuricum acidum for hot flashes followed by trembling and cold sweat-drenching, worse in evening. Valeriana for tightness in throat and chest on dropping to sleep; night cramp in left leg which awakens you; sudden gushes of sweat.

## Dryness and Difficulty with Intercourse

When I was in medical school, we were told that frequent intercourse was the answer to the problem of dryness and difficulty with intercourse: "A well-worn path grows no weeds." Although this may be true, it is difficult to carry through when you're never sure whether it will hurt this time or not. You tense up and try to avoid intercourse or, at best, initiate activity less often. These signals are often misread or not understood by your partner, and distance grows. Yes, this is a common scenario.

Dry eyes, mouth, and nasal passages are less commonly talked about, but they can also be quite troubling. Artificial tears, saline nose sprays and gels, and chewing gum are helpful for these symptoms. For eye dryness, placing freshly cut cucumber slices or wet chamomile tea bags on your eyelids feels very good. Drink lots of water and eat many high-water content fruits and veggies, such as lettuce, melon, cucumber, and spaghetti squash.

HRT, of course, is a specific for all of these ills, but not all women choose this.

Start early (as soon as you read this) with a daily vaginal massage with any good dietary oil. Use oil as a lubricant for lovemaking. (I was once at an airport, scanning the incoming passengers for a family member, when a voice behind me said, "Thanks for the olive oil tip, Michele." Why buy lubricants?) Caution: If you need to use condoms, don't use oils that can break down the rubber. Ditto for diaphragms. Use KY Jelly or another lubricant designed to be used with condoms and diaphragms.

Some women find OstadermV soothing and lubricating. This is Ostaderm in a base that doesn't irritate the tender vulvar and perineal tissues.

A very specific and well-studied solution is estriol vaginal cream. I usually have it compounded in doses of either 2 mg per gram or 5 mg per gram, using the stronger cream (5 mg/gm) in the short term for moderate to severe atrophic vaginitis and the weaker-strength cream for the long term. This is very successful and can be used without fear of causing endometrial cancer.

A dry vagina loses some of its natural protections against infection. Very often intravaginal estriol and/or acidophilus will take care of this, but, if symptoms (itch, pain, and discharge) persist, I suggest that a vaginal culture be done and the specific cause be treated.

Herbal approaches include sitz baths of oat straw and/or comfrey, which are soothing to tender, dry tissues, as are ointments made from comfrey, calendula, and/or wild yam. Lubricating and massaging the vagina with flax seed oil, especially one containing vitamin E, is helpful.

Some people advocate intravaginal acidophilus capsules. I feel this is not a great idea in the absence of any true vaginitis. Obviously, the phytoestrogenic herbs, such as black cohosh, motherwort, and Dong Quai, can be very helpful.

Homeopathic remedies for dryness include Belladonna, Bryonia, and Natrum mur. Belladonna is for dry, hot mouth and throat, while Bryonia is for dry, parched, cracked lips; dry mouth; tongue very dry and rough and coated in the center; bitter taste; dry mucous membranes; and scanty sticky secretions. Cantharis is for raw, inflamed, burning thirst but with an aversion to liquids; scalding urine; sexual irritation. Lycopodium is for sour taste; painful intercourse; dry skin and vagina; rawness in vulva and anus. Natrum mur (sea salt) is for dryness of skin, mouth, throat, rectum, and vagina; thirst; genital herpes; painful intercourse.

## Decreased Libido

Use of estrogen or phytoestrogenic herbs—or both—may be all that's needed to boost libido in many women, but for some women this is not enough. This is where we consider androgens, or male hormones.

DHEA, the current popular "cure-all," is a mildly androgenic adrenal hormone, which in physiologic doses of 10 mg to 15 mg may be sufficient for the woman whose levels are low. (I measure by testing blood or saliva.) Otherwise, the "hormone of desire," to borrow a phrase from Dr. Susan Rako, is testosterone. I have reservations about the commonly prescribed oral preparations, like Estratest, because of the possibility of liver damage with prolonged use. Instead, I prescribe natural testosterone (generic) as a transdermal cream or gel or as a sublingual tablet or a trochee, or methyltestosterone (a synthetic testosterone that does not convert to estradiol) as a cream to be applied directly to the vulvae.

A wild card that needs to be considered when using natural testosterone is that some of it will be converted in the liver, skin, and fat to estradiol, and that each woman does this at her own rate. Because of this, I advocate monitoring levels of testosterone and estradiol when using these preparations. With methyltestosterone, this conversion is less significant and therefore less worrying.

## Dizziness

Usually, the complaint of dizziness is really light-headedness rather than true vertigo, but occasionally episodes of true vertigo may be experienced.

Very often, on discussion, it becomes apparent that eating habits or lifestyle are causing this problem. Usually, remembering to go not longer than three hours without eating something, and making sure that you eat a combination of complex carbohydrate with protein (e.g., an apple wedge with a smear of peanut butter), will take care of the problem. Some busy and absent-minded souls (like me) may even need to set an alarm to remember to do this.

Being too busy and overcommitted can also lead to light-headedness. This is a time of intense inward activity and physiologic change. Pace yourself. Match the rhythm of your life to your breathing: you cannot breathe in without breathing out, and vice versa. Yoga can help.

The herbal suggestions of the scent of lavender oil or drinking primula flower tea are offered in herbal books on menopause, but I have no experience with them. The suggestion to breathe into your cupped hands will, of course, help if you are hyperventilating at all.

I do have personal experience of using the homeopathic remedy Cocculus indicans and have found it usually very helpful, both for lightheadedness and for true vertigo.

## Formication

Formication is an unusual symptom, experienced by approximately 6 to 10 percent of menopausal women. As I said in Chapter 1, formication is a sensation of ants crawling on your skin or, more broadly, an itching or a crawling sensation, usually, but not always, confined to a single area of the body. There will be nothing to see unless you've scratched it raw! I had a six-inch strip on my left forearm that itched mercilessly for two months.

This is a high-class nuisance, but it is not illness. All the suggestions given for dryness are helpful, as are topical anti-itch creams or gels. Cold helps, too.

Homeopathic aids are Caladium, which helps if the itching is in the genital area, and Rhus tox, which is reputed to be helpful for a crawling sensation on the skin.

## Palpitations

Palpitations are actually fairly common at this time and usually do not imply illness, but, to be on the safe side, check with your physician. Most commonly, I find that tincture of reassurance and relaxation does much to alleviate this symptom, and I recommend fifteen to twenty minutes of meditation each morning and a relaxing bedtime ritual. Turn off the stimuli. Beyond this, supplemental magnesium is very helpful, and a dose of 250 to 500 mg usually does the trick.

Herbal preparations that are cardiotonic (soothing to the heart) are hawthorne, motherwort, valerian, and black haw. They have helpful relaxant properties.

Hawthorne appears to have a beneficial effect on minor arrhythmias by improving energy metabolism and the utilization of oxygen in heart muscle. It reduces the accumulation of lactic acid in heart muscle. It is regarded as very low toxicity.

Motherwort (botanical name *Leonardus cardiaca*) has a long history of use in treating hormonal-driven and anxiety-driven rapid heartbeat.

Valerian brings to my mind the Victorian "vapors." Pharmacologically, its effects help to normalize the nervous system and probably help palpitations through a sedative effect and perhaps by decreasing adrenergic drive. It is regarded as safe when using standardized extracts in recommended doses.

Black haw also acts as a sedative and relaxant.

Homeopathic remedies are Spigelia, which is reported to be helpful, especially when palpitations are combined with eye symptoms, such as left eye pain, radiating from the left side of the back of the skull, or swollen, aching eyes; and Rock Rose (Bach flower), which is useful when there is fear and anxiety.

# CHAPTER 6

# Therapeutic Approaches in Postmenopause

## *Urethritis and Cystitis*

Many women develop urethritis and cystitis (infections of the urethra and bladder) as the urethral mucosa loses its hormonal protection. These infections can cause pain or burning during urination, a need to urinate frequently, and low-back pain. (The *urethral mucosa* is the mucous lining of the *urethra*, the tube that transports urine from the bladder to the outside of the body.)

To help prevent infections, it is very important to avoid holding urine—you should schedule your toileting so that you go every three to four hours during the day. And you should *double void*—at the end of the stream, when you think you're done, squeeze again and get the last few drops of any residual urine (you may be unaware that anything more is there until you squeeze). Urine remaining in the bladder can create a breeding ground for bacteria.

Additional protection against these infections includes drinking lots of fluids, taking vitamin C, and using topical estrogens or hormone replacement therapy (if necessary). And, remember, *Don't hold it!* If you have to go, you have to go. Any dammed-up stream can become turbid (translation: any backed-up urine can create conditions that can lead to infection). If urinary symptoms persist, a urine culture and sensitivity should be done to identify what organism is causing an infection, so the appropriate antibiotics can be started.

Herbal remedies for urinary symptoms can be helpful and may make it unnecessary to use antibiotics. Cranberries have been widely held to be helpful in urinary tract infections, and millions of gallons of cranberry juice have been consumed for this purpose. Cranberries were originally thought to be helpful because they acidify the urine. Now we know that both cranberries and blueberries contain a compound that inhibits the ability of bacteria to adhere to the wall of the bladder. Gel caps containing a concentrate of dried cranberries can be purchased, and there are many delicious ways to consume these berries, as well. A dessert can combine cranberries, blueberries, and a little sweetener (I use honey) in a pie, crisp, or cobbler.

Uva ursi has been shown to help clean the urinary tract of microorganisms and is a mild diuretic, clearing urine from the body. It is not as effective as cranberries, however, and it works best in an alkaline urine, which means that you should avoid acid fruits and vitamin C if you're taking uva ursi. Because it is high in tannin content, uva ursi tea should be prepared as "sun tea" (beginning with cold, not hot, water, and brewed in sunlight).

Although echinacea has been used extensively by herbalists to treat a multitude of infectious illnesses, it actually has relatively weak antimicrobial properties and seems to have its major effect by enhancing the immune response. Mallow is a demulcent (a soothing substance used to relieve pain in irritated mucous surfaces) and acts as an anti-inflammatory for mucous membranes. It is soothing but not curative. Yarrow has mild urinary antiseptic properties.

A homeopathic remedy is Cantharis, which is for symptoms of burning, scalding urine; intolerable urgency; bladder spasms; and inability to hold the urine.

## Stress Incontinence

Stress incontinence means involuntarily leaking small or large amounts of urine, often when coughing, sneezing, laughing, or lifting a bundle. Stress incontinence inconveniences many women, often from the time of first pregnancy, although women who have not had children also develop stress incontinence.

The best offense against stress incontinence is Kegel exercises. Kegel, Kegel, Kegel—you cannot do these exercises too often, and they are incredibly helpful. Draw the muscles of your vagina upward and squeeze. Practice turning your urinary stream on and off this way. Physical therapists can be wonderful resources. Some of them teach pelvic floor exercises, to strengthen the muscles that control the flow of urine. Deborah Burnham, a P.T. who works with me, sometimes recommends holding a smooth, rounded clean object in the vagina as a way of testing the strength of your muscles. If you can go about your daily chores, including your more active ones, and not drop this object, you have good muscle tone!

Acupuncture and biofeedback are other approaches that can be helpful. There is now a biofeedback chair, designed specifically for treating stress incontinence.

Estrogen helps tone the pelvic supports. If incontinence is a woman's primary complaint, I generally suggest estriol vaginal cream together with the above suggestions.

One of my favorite tricks, or "medical pearls," is to fit a woman with a diaphragm. She then cuts away the rubber cup and inserts the diaphragm ring upon awakening and takes it out when she goes to bed. The effect is similar to the effect of wearing a pessary (a doughnut-shaped device that is placed inside the vagina by a physician), but wearing the diaphragm is entirely within the woman's control. This has even made it possible for some of my patients to continue their aerobics classes. It does work very well.

In the late 1990s, the Reliance device came on the market. In essence this is a urinary plug that a woman inserts into her urethra. It is similar to a urinary catheter in design, except that it is solid rather than a hollow tube. It is kept in place by a small balloon that inflates at the neck of the bladder and blocks urinary flow. Somehow, I doubt that any woman who has ever been catheterized will be eager to try this, and it has not become popular. In medical school, I was taught that the most common cause of scarring and stricture of the urethra is insertion of a foreign body—usually a catheter. Catheters also commonly cause infection and I can't imagine that our experience with this device will be any different. Reliance is available by prescription and comes in five sizes.

Surgery is always an option for stress incontinence, but I think it's best as an option, not the first choice. Most of my patients do not end up having surgery.

Avoid bladder irritants like caffeine, smoking, and the following foods, if they give you trouble: apple juice, carbonated drinks, coffee, vinegar, cranberries, guava, peaches, plums, onions, apples, cantaloupe, chilies/spicy foods, strawberries, grapes, lemon, pineapple, tomato, alcoholic beverages.

Herbally, black cohosh can be helpful in the same way that any estrogen source is, that is, by toning and moisturizing the involved tissues. Catnip is listed as helpful because of its reputed antispasmodic qualities. In his book *Holistic Herbal*, David Hoffman describes the benefits of a mixture of horsetail, agrimony, and sweet sumach.

Homeopathic remedies for stress incontinence include Causticum, Ferrum phos. (phosphoricum), and Pulsatilla. Causticum is the choice for loss of control with coughing and sitting, and for dribbling during urination. Pulsatilla is useful for nighttime incontinence, accompanied by a heavy bearing-down sensation in the bladder. Ferrum phos. applies when you have to pee after every drink—or maybe even at the thought of drinking.

## Hypertension

A woman may develop hypertension, or high blood pressure, as the tone of the blood vessels diminishes in response to reduced amounts of estrogen. Recent studies have shown that within half an hour of an estrogen dose, the peripheral blood vessels dilate, or open wider. This improves blood flow and would tend to lower blood pressure. Indeed, I have observed a lowering of blood pressure in some patients after they use an estrogen source, but we must be cautious about this.

Lifestyle can be very important and, certainly, weight loss is important here. Given a choice between weight loss and smoking cessation, however, I would say quit smoking first and then focus on the weight. Also, I wouldn't "diet," but would instead keep my focus on eating for health. This means lots of fruits and vegetables. Ten or eleven servings of fruit and vegetables consumed daily can reduce blood pressure all by themselves (see Appendix 1). Ensuring adequate calcium, magnesium, and potassium intake is important, as well. Plant foods help ensure adequate potassium intake. You can take a calcium/magnesium supplement and consume dairy products, kidney beans, peanut butter, kale, spinach, and beet greens to ensure the intake of these important minerals.

Exercise is important for many reasons and is necessary to

help metabolism and general body toning, but exercise alone has not been demonstrated to lower blood pressure.

In the 1970s, studies on Transcendental Meditation showed that meditation can lower blood pressure. Certainly it is one of the most powerful stress reducers and can be done by anyone. Meditation is not a "New Age" technique or a foreign (that is, Eastern) idea. The practice of meditation exists in all religious and philosophical traditions and is foreign only to our fast-paced, goal-oriented current culture. My grandfather saying his rosary every night before bed, sitting quietly, erectly, in the dark, was, in effect, meditating. Knitting can be a form of meditation. Being totally aware and present in the moment can be a meditation. Meditation can be devotional, but it need not be. Try it!

The most valuable herb for high blood pressure is hawthorne. It is mild and requires time, sometimes as long as two weeks, to show any effect. Like the well-known drugs Capoten, Vasotec, and Lotensin, hawthorne acts in a number of ways: it inhibits angiotensin-converting enzymes and acts as a tonic on heart muscle. It also dilates the blood vessels, like the drug Minipres, and has a very mild diuretic action. In studies, it has repeatedly been shown to lower blood pressure.

Garlic is a valuable tool in lowering blood pressure. Indeed, studies have shown a systolic decrease of about 20 mm Hg and a diastolic of about 15. I see no reason not to use both hawthorne and standardized extract of garlic (900 mg daily). Also, increase your dietary use of garlic and cook with a lot of onion.

Motherwort is a source of phytoestrogen and is reputed to have a tonic effect on the cardiovascular system. Dandelion, especially as a tea or beverage, is a very helpful diuretic, especially as it is rich in potassium and will not deplete you, as many diuretics do.

## Fractures and Bone Pain

Fractures and bone pain were covered in the section of Chapter 2 discussing osteoporosis, but not all the herbal and homeopathic remedies were discussed there. I also want to say again that you don't know the status of your bones unless you have a bone density measurement. This test is now much easier to obtain because most insurers now cover it, following the lead of Medicare. Beginning in July 1998, all Medicare patients at risk of osteoporosis are covered for a bone density measurement every two years. Also, as far as I know, there is no truly reliable nonhormonal, nondrug way to treat established osteoporosis.

Herbal allies in preventing fractures and bone pain are horsetail, wild yam, and skullcap. Horsetail tea is a source of minerals, especially in combination with calcium-rich herbs like dandelion. Wild yam cream can be a source of progesterone. Some studies show that progesterone has a bone-building effect and that it augments this effect in estrogen. Skullcap is supposed to act by relaxing muscle, and it may relieve pain in this way.

Homeopathic allies in preventing fractures and bone pain include Arnica, Silica, and Ruta. Arnica, topically applied, as well as sublingually (under the tongue), is used for relief of the feeling of bruised soreness. Cuprum met. (metallicum) is indicated for cramping, spastic pain, especially at night. Nux vomica is for a bruised feeling shot through with stabbing pains. Rhus tox is for shooting, tearing pains accompanied by stiffness, which is worst at night. Ruta is for pain deep in the long bones, relieved by walking, and when bones are brittle. Silica is for painful sensitivity to cold, with pain in the arch of the foot.

Let us not neglect the value of safety in the home: take away any area rugs that may trip you. Avoid slick, wet floors. No loose electrical cords on the floor. Install hand grips and railings in the bathrooms and stairwells. Forget high heels! Analyze your home for safety.

TENS, or transcutaneous (*cutaneous* = skin) electrical nerve stimulation, can be helpful for bone pain. To use this, you connect electrodes to two, three, or four points on your body and then the electrodes are connected to a battery pack worn at your waist. The TENS device provides little "shocks" that help with the pain. How TENS works is not well understood— but it often does provide significant relief from pain.

## Foot and Leg Cramps and Twitchiness

Legs that feel in constant motion, with or without pain in the legs or feet, can disturb your rest as effectively as any megawatt "power surge." In my experience, these symptoms most commonly signal a need for increased calcium, magnesium, or vitamin E, or some combination of these. If you are obtaining these minerals and vitamin E in adequate amounts but your legs are still dancing, a glass or two of tonic water, which contains quinine, usually does the trick. Only rarely have I needed to prescribe quinine sulfate.

For an herbal approach, sprinkle oil of peppermint or rosemary into a hot bath and have a lovely soak before bed. (Nice even if you don't have a problem with leg cramps.) Or try black haw, which acts as an antispasmodic and sedative, or St. John's wort, which has sedative, anti-inflammatory and pain-relieving properties.

Homeopathic remedies for foot and leg cramps and twitchiness include Arsenicum when the sensation is like burning hot needles in the feet and legs. Chamomilla is the choice when the legs feel restless, with or without spasms. Cuprum matches with true cramps and muscle spasms in the feet and legs. Nux vomica is particularly indicated for brunettes experiencing tenderness in the legs with stabbing spasms.

## Wrinkles and Droops

Wrinkles and droops, or the ongoing attraction of gravity, happens to all of us to lesser or greater degree (genes play a big role). Personally, I find the bland faces of youth far less interesting than those bearing the scars and citations of life. My life has been full of joy and sorrow; how can I appear unmarked? Rejoice in your smile lines! An unmarked face is an unused one.

Skin's three worst enemies are sun, smoking, and excessive alcohol. Needless to say, now is a little late, but better late than never. We should emulate our grandmothers, who always wore bonnets and carried parasols. Or at least use sunscreen that provides protection from both UVA and UVB rays.

A healthy diet is the skin's best ally. This means plenty of water, fruits and vegetables, and essential fatty acids.

Many products are available to help keep skin youthful. The skin creams containing retinoids, alpha hydroxyacids, and/or antioxidants all do, indeed, help to smooth out the skin and improve its tone. Vitamin E creams may be beneficial. Most are available without prescription. And, yes, hormone replacement therapy does help the skin stay youthful.

Face lifts and chemical peels are easily available and are part of the vast industry catering to the pursuit of everlasting youth. These are painful, expensive, and potentially hazardous procedures. I hope that you will soul search very deeply before submitting yourself to these techniques.

For sags and bags under the eyes, a tip given me by air hostesses is to carefully apply over-the-counter hemorrhoid cream! It works well (unless, like me, you react to it with a rash). Herbal allies are creams made of sage, nettle, and wild yam. A cucumber slice over puffy eyes is soothing and reduces puffiness.

# CHAPTER 7

# Estriol
## The Forgotten Estrogen

When I finally had the insight that I was menopausal, I was faced with the same choices as my patients. Initially I used a variety of lifestyle and herbal approaches, but I found that, for me, it was not possible to devote the time necessary for successful self-care without sacrificing family or patient time. This was not an option, not only because of the practicalities but because service is where I personally find satisfaction. Also, I seemed to be truly blocked in my ability to center myself, making meditation very difficult. Gregorian chant and Celtic harp became my allies in this search for centering. I was now awakening every hour every night and never felt rested or in control.

So, what to do? My family had breast cancer on both sides, both pre- and postmenopausal. Mom had shrunk a couple of inches. My lipid profile had always been very good, but I needed thyroid medication for hypothyroidism. The pros and cons. Confusion.

Desperation for sleep decided the matter. With the idea that I could always change my mind, I bagan to take estriol in capsule form. By the second day, I was sleeping again.

As every medical student learns, *estrogen* is a generic term for a hormone that comes in several varieties. Women produce three main types of estrogens: estradiol (or E2), estrone (or E1), and estriol (or E3). Estradiol is the predominant estrogen produced by the ovaries, and it dominates during our menstruating years. It is the type most commonly thought of as "estrogen." Estrone is produced from estradiol in the liver. Estrone is the dominant estrogen during our postmenopausal years, because it is stored in and produced by our fatty tissues. This is why some heavy postmenopausal women have more estrogenic effect on their tissues than some very thin women who are still in their late thirties. Both estrone and estradiol are associated with higher risks of breast and endometrial cancer. Indeed, estrogen supplementation with estrone or estradiol will cause a 12 percent incidence of endometrial cancer in users. This risk is nullified when estrone or estradiol is combined with progesterone. (The risk in the general population of women *not* taking estrone or estradiol is less than 1 percent.) Because the risk of breast and endometrial cancer increases after menopause, one cannot help but wonder if there could be a causal link with estrone.

Estriol is the dominant estrogen of pregnancy and accounts for about 10 percent of circulating estrogen in a nonpregnant woman. It is basically the detoxification product of estradiol and estrone and, in the pregnant state, is augmented by production by the placenta from fetal DHEA. DHEA (dihydroepiandosterone) is a weak androgen (male hormone) and is an intermediate step in the synthesis of testosterone and progesterone. In pregnancy, the placenta can secrete up to fifty times the amount of total estriol produced by the liver during an average monthly cycle. Our young pregnant women could perhaps sell their urine to a pharmaceutical house, giving the women supplemental income and giving us a rich source of human estrogens! Harebrained? Maybe, maybe not. It seems as feasible as using pregnant mare's urine to make Premarin (a prescription estrogen), and obviously, the technology is available.

There is evidence in the literature that estriol may be not

only noncarcinogenic but perhaps even protective. In countries with lower rates of breast cancer than ours, women have higher average urinary levels of estriol. A 1956 study showed that women with breast cancer had lower urinary levels of estriol than women who did not have breast cancer. A study done by Henry M. Lemon in the 1970s demonstrated dramatic inhibition of breast cancer in mice exposed to carcinogens when these mice were treated with estriol. The study confirmed this same effect in a small group of women with advanced breast cancer. This study was not intended to determine whether estriol could be used as treatment, but rather to assess its safety and effectiveness for menopausal symptoms. It was never published but was referred to in a 1978 article in the *Journal of the American Medical Association*, by A. H. Follingstad.

In a 1993 article in the *New England Journal of Medicine*, R. Raz and Walter Stamm reported that the daily use of estriol vaginal cream prevented urinary tract infections in postmenopausal women who had been plagued by recurrent urinary infections. They also referred to several other papers reporting the same finding and confirming the safety of this approach. These studies indicate that estriol can "juice up" and rejuvenate the vagina and the cervix without causing proliferation of the endometrium (overgrowth of the cells lining the uterus, which can create the precancerous condition known as hyperplasia; see Chapter 2). We do need to be aware that an oral—not a vaginal—estriol has been demonstrated to show an increased risk of uterine cancer (3 percent) in women who use oral estiol daily. The cancers were mostly of low virulence and were not apt to be invasive. This risk was not recognized earlier. As with other estrogen preparations, use of a progesterone negates this risk. Knowledge of the risk allows us to be vigilant in our follow-up of anyone using estriol orally.

In a 1976 paper published in *Acta Obstetrica et Gynaecologica Scandinavia*, C. Lauritzen advocated treatment of menopausal symptoms when they cause suffering to women. He compared the efficacy of 2 mg of estriol daily with 1.25 mg of conjugated equine estrogens in the relief of hot flashes, sweating, vertigo, palpitations, irritability, anxiety, insomnia, depression, and headache. He found that estriol was at least as good at relieving most symptoms and was better for insomnia and headache. He also demonstrated that it was safer than conjugated equine estrogen in terms of endometrial proliferation.

Here in the United States, estriol has indeed been the forgotten estrogen. There is a common misperception that it is too weak to be effective, even though basic biochemistry and physiology textbooks state that the weaker estrogens, such as estriol, are potent if dosed frequently and adequately. Lauritzen's study provides a good guideline for proper dosing, and my own experience with it over the past ten years has been gratifying in terms of results.

When I first started prescribing estriol, I had a quandary: was it effective in preventing osteoporosis and in lowering lipid levels? My gut sense was yes, since it certainly relieved menopausal symptoms, but it wouldn't be right to blindly give this assurance to my patients. This became part of our dialogue, and the resultant plan was that we would track bone densities and lipid levels so we could use other early interventions if estriol wasn't doing the job. At the time, virtually no insurers were paying for bone density studies (thankfully, this has changed), but these women were committed to trying what was probably a safer way through menopause.

Sofia is a good example. Sofia is a tall, willowy blond whom I first saw when she was forty-three. It would be difficult to have a healthier lifestyle than she; she's a health care provider who eats a well-balanced vegetarian diet, exercises regularly, teaches yoga, and meditates daily. She is a very well informed woman who could not tolerate her night sweats and insomnia—the fatigue was interfering with her professional life and the vaginal dryness with her personal life. For many reasons, Sofia was opposed to using estrogen. We discussed all of the options and agreed on the helpfulness of a bone density measurement and lipid studies. As expected, her cholesterol and HDL were great. But, much to our dismay, Sofia was already osteoporotic! What to do?

After much discussion and thought, Sofia opted for estriol at a dose of 2 mg daily. She also increased her calcium intake in the form of calcium hydroxyapatite with boron. She was still having her menses, so we decided to wait to add progesterone. Six weeks later, Sofia came in, beaming, and said "Michele, my body says thank you, thank you, thank you." Two years later, Sofia and I had even more reason for happiness: her repeat bone density showed an 11 percent improvement.

Dixie entered my office looking like a starved refugee. When she told me that one year earlier she had been a very active woman with a full teaching load and psychotherapy practice, I quite truthfully had reservations as to how that could be. During the previous year, Dixie had been diagnosed with major depression, chronic fatigue syndrome, and fibromyalgia, and she was now on total disability. She was having difficulty maintaining a weight of ninety pounds, had limp, dull, dry hair, dry skin, and an exceedingly vulnerable "feel." Dixie is an astute woman and was sure that her endocrine system was involved in her collapse. As usual, we agreed first to try simple things that might not help but wouldn't harm in the trying.

For Dixie, this plan consisted of adjusting her dose of thyroid medication; adding milled flax seed to her diet; making her diet more colorful with veggies and fruits; and beginning on oral estriol. Dixie was also agonizing over a long-term relationship that had lost its fizz; her partner was incredibly supportive and she felt that she loved him, but she wasn't sure that the relationship was promoting her self-growth. I suggested that she put major decisions on hold until she felt more able, and I asked her to keep a color journal—each day to draw or paint an entry of whatever colors she felt moved to use. We agreed not to change her antidepressant medication.

Three months later, I returned to the office after lunch one day and Gail said to me, "Dixie's in the waiting room."

"Really? I only saw the new patient," I responded.

When I went back to the waiting room, its sole occupant, a very attractive woman with springy reddish curls, looked up and smiled. "It's me, Michele."

Today, Dixie has her estriol prescription written by her HMO doctor, and I hear news of her through the many clients and friends she refers, who are as amazed and overjoyed by her transformation as am I.

Do all women respond like Sofia and Dixie? No, each woman is unique and, if this is appreciated, her needs can be met.

Sameea is a slip of a woman: wiry, dark-haired, dark-eyed, forty-five, and previously a dynamo. She loves the outdoors and had recently moved from a large city to the mountains. Shortly after she moved, she was suddenly exhausted all the time; over the next few months, she noticed she had no interest in sex and was forgetting things at work. Initially, Sameea chalked all this up to the stress of a move and a new job, but then the hot flashes started—with a vengeance! And then, the period-skipping.

Sameea's friend Sally lives in New Hampshire and is a patient of mine. Sally invited Sameea to come visit and to have an appointment with me. Sameea had already been utilizing all the nonpharmaceutical approaches and was still "flashing" every hour. Her nights were torments. By then, she had not cycled for six months.

The first dose of estriol that I prescribed for Sameea gave her several nights of good sleep and greatly diminished "flashing." Within a week, however, we were back to square one. When she phoned me, I suggested she try a dose at breakfast and another at 6 P.M., thereby doubling her initial small doses and extending its action. Two weeks later, this was reported as much better, but not yet perfect. In response to this, I asked our pharmacist, George Roentsch, to make up a dose two and a half times the original dose, and to time-release it over twenty-four hours. So far, so good!

It's been my observation that when women are in the throes of hormonal turbulence, they may actually require more supplemental hormone than they will when they become postmenopausal. The literature cites doses of up to 20 mg of estriol. Frequently, though, I will use a very small dose of estradiol for its greater potency and longer half-life in addition to estriol, if stabilization on estriol alone becomes too frustrating or too expensive. Estriol is almost always the predominant estrogen that I prescribe.

A woman may also report changing needs related to her menstrual cycle, if she still cycles regularly. (Or irregularly regularly.) A wonderfully helpful tool in this case is the PMS chart in Chapter 1. Alix is a good example. Most of the month she does fine with 2.5 mg of estriol, but she needs to take an additional 0.5 mg of estriol for seven days before her period starts. Her need clearly shows itself, as she becomes very irritable. And this irritability does not occur in the months when she skips her period.

As mentioned previously, estriol causes very little, if any, proliferation of the endometrium, so there is more latitude in regard to the need to take progesterone along with estriol. As you will remember, in order to protect against the risk of endometrial cancer, conventionally, progesterone must be used together with estrogen in a woman who still has her uterus.

R. B. Greenblatt, M.D., has called progesterone the "unhappy hormone" because it can cause a depressed mood in many women. Many women complain of migraine associated with progesterone use, or of feeling bloated or "PMS-y." A bedtime dosing with progesterone can often take advantage of the "downer" effect and help with sleep. I've found that for most women for whom this fails or who are plagued by progesterone-associated migraines, progesterone can be better tolerated in the form of a transdermal cream, compounded by a pharmacist. When this is used, I usually have the estrogen compounded in the cream in combination with the progesterone. This is primarily for convenience and affordability. Critics question whether this is an effective delivery route, but I have satisfied myself by checking serum or salivary levels of the relevant hormones. Not to mention the effect on symptoms and well-being.

Why use progesterone at all if I'm taking estriol? This is a question I've posed to myself, coming up with two good reasons. First, although estriol undoubtedly affects the uterus less than estradiol or estrone, no studies have yet addressed the effect of long-term use of estriol on the uterine lining. Second, there is evidence that estrogen and progesterone act synergistically in preventing osteoporosis.

It has been stated at conferences and in journal articles that only 30 percent of women prescribed hormone replacement are compliant—that is, take their prescribed hormone medication. Indeed, many of my patients have told me that they have been noncompliant with hormone replacement therapy in the past. From them, I think I know why noncompliance is so high.

Nadine, a strikingly attractive CEO of a financial service company, stated: "He handed me a prescription, told me it was natural and would protect my heart and bones, I should take it the rest of my life, he'd see me next year. And then he was out the door. I went to the drugstore and found out it comes from horse's piss, might cause cancer, and I was going to get my period back. His prescription went in my circular file. Damn it, I'm an intelligent woman, and I know I need to look at these things, but I want to be informed and part of the decision-making process. Tell me my options, define my risks, and let me take responsibility for my decisions."

Nadine is typical of the women I see in that all of them want factual information about what is available and want to know what their own risk factors are and what their health care provider believes to be their best option. Also, every woman wants to be respected if her decision is not in accord with the expressed opinion of the health care provider.

Virtually all of the women in my practice who have chosen to use estriol have been happy with their choice.

# CHAPTER 8

# Hormone Replacement Therapy

When I wrote the first edition of this book, HRT was being prescribed more liberally than vitamin pills. Now, the same doctor who shoved the prescription at Nadine is telling his patients, "You've got to get off your HRT whether you want to or not. I won't be responsible for writing a prescription for it."

In the course of my professional life, I have seen many shifts in medical opinion about the use of hormones, always reflecting the science of the day. My generation were the earliest beneficiaries of, and we served as "point women" (guinea pigs) for, "the Pill" and the sexual freedom it gave us. From the point of view of health, the oral contraceptive has been a great gift to young women, freeing them from the risks inherent in unwanted pregnancies. Bonuses have been a reduced risk of ovarian cancer and a beneficial effect on bone density.

In the 1970s, articles in the medical journals recommended the use of hormones to treat the symptoms of menopause, but prescribing them was frowned on in this country. This was partly because of our fears of breast and uterine cancer and our recent bad experience with DES (diethylstilbestrol, a drug prescribed in the 1940s, 1950s, and 1960s to help a woman carry a pregnancy to term, which eventually was shown to cause cancer in some of the female offspring who had been exposed to the drug in utero, in addition to other problems in both female and male offspring). We were not yet aware of any of the preventive benefits conferred by the use of hormone replacement therapy, nor were we as aware of women's risk of osteoporosis as we are today.

In the 1990s, the trend again went to the extreme, with our belief that estrogen was the elixir of youth for women and would prevent just about all of the degenerative diseases suffered by modern women. Yes, we acknowledged that there is a slight increase in incidence of breast cancer among women using HRT, but all the other benefits outweighed this risk. Initial results from several large studies indicated that use of HRT reduced the overall mortality from all cancers, including breast cancer. So why not put it in the drinking water?

Now, in our second millennium, with more studies and more statistics, the pendulum has again swung. Doctors are quickly backpedaling to take women off their hormones, lest someone sue them, and women are panicking at media accounts stating that use of HRT is associated with a 26 percent increase in breast cancer, mistakenly thinking this means that each woman has a 26 percent chance of developing breast cancer if she has used HRT. In fact, the risk for any woman who is not at high risk for other reasons (and who therefore shouldn't be using hormones for those reasons) is about 10 percent without HRT; if she uses HRT, that risk increases by about 1/10 percent (one-tenth of one percent) per year of use. Another way of saying this is to recognize that for every 10,000 women, an extra eight cases of invasive breast cancer per year can be blamed on HRT.

We also firmly believed, based on a large number of studies, that estrogen was relatively heart-protective. From the most recent studies, it is clear that women aged 65 and older who already have coronary heart disease are at increased risk of worsening this disease on HRT especially in the first year of taking HRT.

What options are available in FDA-approved hormones?

## Table 6. Estrogens, Progestins, and Combinations

| Type or Trade Name | Method of Administration | Doses | Interval |
|---|---|---|---|
| ESTROGENS | | | |
| *Conjugated Equine Estrogens [estrone]* | | | |
| Premarin | oral/vaginal | multiple | daily |
| Cenestin | oral | one | daily |
| *Esterified Estrogens [estrone]* | | | |
| Estratab | oral | multiple | daily |
| Menest | oral | multiple | daily |
| *17-β-Estradiol* | | | |
| Climara | patch | two | weekly |
| Estrace | oral/vaginal | multiple | daily |
| Vivelle | patch | multiple | twice/week |
| FemPatch | patch | one | weekly |
| Estraderm | patch | two | twice/week |
| Alora | patch | multiple | twice/week |
| Estring | vaginal | one | every 3 mo. |
| Estrasorb | topical | one | daily |
| *Estropipate [estrone]* | | | |
| Ortho-Est | oral | two | daily |
| PROGESTINS | | | |
| *Medroxyprogesterone Acetate* | | | |
| Amen | oral | one | sequential |
| Cycrin | oral | multiple | sequential |
| Provera | oral | multiple | daily/sequential |
| *Norethindrone Acetate* | | | |
| Aygestin | oral | one | daily/sequential |
| *Natural Progesterone* | | | |
| Prometrium | oral | one | daily/sequential |
| Crinone | vaginal | two | sequential |

Table 6. *Estrogens, Progestins, and Combinations* (continued)

| Type or Trade Name | Method of Administration | Doses | Interval |
|---|---|---|---|

COMBINATIONS

*Conjugated Equine Estrogens and Medroxyprogesterone Acetate*

| | | | |
|---|---|---|---|
| Prempro | oral | two | daily |
| Premphase | oral | one | sequential |

*17-β-Estradiol and Norethindrone Acetate*

| | | | |
|---|---|---|---|
| CombiPatch | patch | two | twice/week |
| Climara Pro | patch | two | once/week |

Table 6 lists many of the available choices. (Keeping Table 6 handy may help you to have a more meaningful discussion with your own doctor.)

Let's look closely at Table 6 and discuss the various options. First, what about conjugated equine estrogens? These were the first estrogens commonly used for HRT and are still the most common estrogens prescribed in the United States, although not necessarily in the world. As implied by the name, conjugated equine estrogen (CEE) is of equine—or horse—origin. In fact, it is extracted from the urine of pregnant mares. The dominant fraction of estrogen in CEE is estrone, but it contains many fractions, including some, such as equilin (a horse estrogen), which are foreign to humans. Very many of the studies investigating the risks and benefits of estrogen have been based on CEE, which conveys all of the benefits we have talked about. Let me summarize them again:

Benefits of estrogen
1. Increases HDL (good cholesterol)
2. Decreases LDL (bad cholesterol)
3. Protects against osteoporosis and decreases the risk of fractures

4. Decreases colon cancer risk
5. May decrease the risk of Alzheimers' disease
6. May slow the progression of Parkinson's disease
7. May counteract some risks of type-2 diabetes
8. Keeps skin youthful
9. Imparts feelings of well-being
10. Keeps vagina moist
11. Ameliorates menopausal symptoms

Risks of hormone replacement

1. Increased risk of breast cancer
2. Increased severity of cardiovascular disease in women who already have cardiovascular disease
3. Increased risk of blood clots

CEE is available in a variety of doses. Recently Wyeth, the manufacturers of Prempro, the most popular combination in the United States brought out a step-down dose of .45g Premarin/1.5g Provera, in hopes that this will be safer than the standard regimen. It is often used to wean women from the higher does.

Even before the current scare, many women did not like CEE. Many object to the use of equine estrogens, some from an animal cruelty point of view, some from an aesthetic point of view (they don't like the idea of it). Others have noted unpleasant side effects like nausea, headache, mood changes and breakthrough bleeding (bleeding when you are not having a period).

The esterified estrogens (of plant origin) are primarily estrone, and much to my surprise, also have equilin added to them. I am not sure what the rationale for this is, especially as there have been at least a couple of hints in the literature that equilin may contribute to the increased breast cancer risk. The esterified estrogens are similar to the conjugated equine estrogens but may be better tolerated, probably because the molecular structure of the plant-derived estrogens is bioidentical to the molecules of estrogen that we make ourselves. (*Bioidentical* means that the molecule is identical to the human molecule.) A number of studies have found that women have fewer side effects on the plant-derived hormones and are therfore happier with them.

Seventeen-$\beta$-estradiol is a plant-derived estrogen. Recall that estradiol is the fraction of estrogen that dominates during our menstruating years, is the most potent, and has the longest half-life. Remember Sameea from Chapter 7? When last I spoke of her, she was doing reasonably well on estriol, but that was short-lived. Eventually, Sameea and I came to the consensus that estriol just wasn't going to "cut it" for her, and now she is happily using one of the transdermal patches of estradiol. This has worked much better for her, primarily, I think, because of its long half-life. Because 17-$\beta$-estradiol is plant-derived and identical to the human molecule, it satisfies Sameea's deisre to use only "natural" hormones.

Let's take a brief detour and look at what we mean by *natural*. Technically, most of the available forms of hormone replacement therapy are natural. What could be more natural than horses' urine? But this is not what women mean in this context: they mean natural *to us*. As mentioned before, the plant-derived hormones fit this bill because they are bioidentical to ours. In fact, several studies have shown the plant-derived estrogens to be better tolerated and more effective in relieving hot flashes and emotional symptoms than equine estrogens.

Seventeen-β-estradiol is available in oral form (pill), in transdermal patches, and in a topical form. More about the patches soon.

In October 2003, the FDA approved the first topical, non-patch, estrogen replacement therapy. It was specifically approved for the hot flashes and night sweats that plague many women. This new product, called Estrasorb, is an emulsion of 17-β-estradiol packaged in single dose pouches, each of which supplies one day's dose of estrogen. You apply the contents of the pouch to your upper leg once daily. The absorption peaks at about twelve to eighteen hours and has been shown to be effective in reducing the number and intensity of hot flashes and night sweats. Like the patch, this approach provides transdermal absorption, which has been shown in many recent studies to be safer than taking estrogen orally.

Estropipate (Ortho-Est) is also a plant-derived estrogen, but it is essentially estrone. Ogen, which is no longer available in the United States, was another brand of estropipate.

We've already discussed the down sides to taking estrogen, but let me reiterate that there is an increased risk of breast cancer, and of breast cancer deaths, associated with HRT use, there is a worsening of cardiovascular disease in women with pre-existing coronary artery disease, and there is an increased risk of blood clots, so that anyone who has ever had a deep vein thrombosis or a pulmonary embolus should not even think about HRT. An interesting finding in several recent studies is that these risks are lower—although still present—in women whose hormone is delivered through the skin and not swallowed. There is also a breath of hope for women who do not want to give up their HRT in the findings from the Women's Health Initiative study that ibuprofen, in a dose of at least 200 mg per week, reduces the risk of breast cancer by 49 percent, with no difference between those women using HRT and those not. Aspirin, in a dose of at least 325 mg per week, reduced the risk by 21 percent. So why would anyone not take ibuprofen or aspirin? There is still very much for us to learn about all of this.

Another side effect may be migraine headaches for women who are prone to migraines. I have found in practice that the culprit is more often the progestin than the estrogen component of the HRT and, indeed, at the 2003 meeting of the American Headache Society, it was announced that use of transdermal estradiol may be helpful in preventing migraine. This study needs to be confirmed by larger-scale studies.

There is also an increased risk of gallstones and gallbladder disease in women using HRT. And an increase in asthma. Last but far from least, estrogen causes up to a 12 percent risk of endometrial (uterine) cancer; in the general population the risk is less than 1 percent.

And that brings us to progesterone. The use of progesterone together with estrogen, in a woman who has her uterus, will protect that woman from the added risk of endometrial cancer. In fact, the resulting risk is actually lower than the risk for the woman who takes no hormones whatsoever. This is truly impressive. What other good things can progesterone do for you?

1. If taken at bedtime, the depressant of progesterone can translate to a calming, sedating one and help you sleep.
2. It can augment the action of estrogen in preventing hot flashes.
3. It enhances the libido, especially together with testosterone.
4. It augments the protective action of estrogen on bone.

Medroxyprogesterone acetate is the most widely used progestin in the United States. In fact, many doctors are unaware of other forms of progesterone. This is too bad, because medroxyprogesterone acetate (the most common brand name is Provera) has some very significant disadvantages. First of all, many women do not feel well on it. They complain of feeling "PMS-y," depressed, and headachy. Altogether quite unpleasant. It also blocks the beneficial effect of estrogen on HDL, the good cholesterol, and the ability of estrogen to dilate blood vessels. I have never understood why it has been so widely prescribed.

Norethindrone acetate is prescribed much less often. It offers some slight advantage over medroxyprogesterone acetate. In studies, its effect on the blood fats was more neutral.

Until the past fifteen years, natural progesterone was only available in very messy suppositories because the crystalline form of it was not very well absorbed by the oral route and was rapidly converted in the liver. The advent of the process of micronization changed all that, and oral micronized progesterone is well absorbed and is available to the body. It has distinct advantages over other forms of progesterone in that it is better tolerated (it is much less likely to cause PMS symptoms), it does not interfere with the effects of estrogen on the blood fats, does not raise blood pressure, and it is safe in early pregnancy (now, isn't that just what you wanted to hear?). Prometrium was approved by the FDA in 1998 and is widely available.

Crinone is a natural progesterone vaginal gel. It comes in a 4 percent and an 8 percent dosage. A dosage of one applicator of 8 percent gel once a day or 4 percent twice daily for ten to fourteen days is the approved usage. This will induce withdrawal bleeding or a "period." It has most commonly been used in treating infertility, but it is useful for women who don't tolerate oral progestins. Soon a similar vaginal gel will be available that is indicated for our stage of life.

Now we have the *what*, let's talk about the *how*. There are two basic ways to prescribe hormone replacement therapy: sequential therapy and continuous therapy. *Sequential therapy means* that you take estrogen for all or most of the cycle and add progesterone for the last ten to fourteen days. You then stop the progesterone and have a "period." (This is in quotes because it is not really a natural period but rather *withdrawal bleeding.* Withdrawal bleeding is purely stimulated by the progesterone and does not imply ovulation or any risk of pregnancy. In my practice, only three women have desired to continue having "periods.") *Continuous therapy* means that you take a very small dose of progesterone together with your daily estrogen and you do not have withdrawal bleeding. Both ways are equally protective of the endometrium. There are a number of ways to vary both of these approaches, all of them equally acceptable.

Combination patches, such as CombiPatch, are not as popular in the United States as they are in Europe, but with the newer studies indicating that transdermal delivery of hormone is safer, patches may gain in popularity. Because they combine the estrogen and the progestin in the same patch, they are very convenient. I was introduced to these patches by a good friend from Dublin, Ireland, who came to visit one Thanksgiving. Her doctor prescribed the CombiPatch for her not long before her visit. He instructed her to leave it off for one week of each month so she would have a withdrawal bleed. Her comment? "Ah, jaysus, Michele, the hot flashes are brutal during that week. And I thought I was all done with that business!" You don't need to leave the patch off for a week, but can use this delivery method continuously.

We used to think that we might not get as much benefit from transdermal estrogen because the estrogen didn't pass through the liver and affect the blood fats in the same way as oral estrogen. Recent studies indicate that transdermal delivery of estrogen poses a much reduced risk of breast cancer, endometrial cancer, and blood clots than does oral estrogen, however.

Perhaps in the future we will have a vaginal mode of delivery for hormone replacement, with a combination of estrogen and progesterone. Such a mode of delivery for birth control is already available.

I have tried to present this information on HRT in an objective way, as I am neither a proponent nor an opponent of hormone replacement therapy. In life there are no guarantees, and everything I can think of carries both benefits and risks. It is not my place to make decisions for readers but rather to provide information so they can make their own informed decisions. You are the one who must live with your decision (and don't forget that you can change your mind, too.)

# Conclusion
## Vision and Responsibility

Most of the physical discomforts of the menopausal process are transient and can be eased using a combination of the therapeutic approaches described in the pages of this book. The drive toward completeness of self can be a lasting legacy of this process.

Today we are often given the message that the spiritual quest or search for fulfillment of one's highest self is at odds with the path of duty and responsibility that so often claims us as women. Certainly, the easier path often is not the path of commitment to the promises made in life. We are often encouraged to value only those people or situations that "allow us to grow," and we fail to learn the lessons of patience, humility, tolerance, and kindness. Nor do we appreciate how these differ from resignation, defeat, and low self-esteem. We are spiritual beings, and our paths are many and diverse. It demeans us to limit ourselves to the path of greatest comfort or popularity or ease. Remaining ever mindful and attentive to the pull to the light, and cherishing an inner quiet and centeredness, will allow us to flourish in many circumstances.

As postmenopausal women, crones, and wise women, we have a very special energy. My observation has been that our caretaking role shifts from the intensely personal and intimate to a more detached and global one. I don't know if this was always true, and certainly it is not true of every woman, but it is true of oh, so many women I see. We are the Grandmothers of the Earth, guarding its wisdom and directing our collective energy toward healthy change, toward a sustainable balance in our ecosystem. We are on each continent, in every country, and our numbers increase each day. We are powerful. We are the Keepers of the Vision of Peace and Abundance for All. The vision is held and spoken and, being spoken, takes form. For these reasons, we need to take care of ourselves.

# Diets for Improved Health and Fitness

*Mediterranean Diet Pyramid*

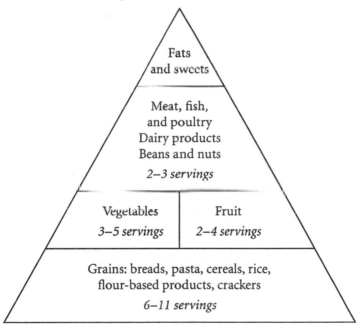

Fats
and sweets

Meat, fish,
and poultry
Dairy products
Beans and nuts

*2–3 servings*

Vegetables

*3–5 servings*

Fruit

*2–4 servings*

Grains: breads, pasta, cereals, rice,
flour-based products, crackers

*6–11 servings*

The Mediterranean Pyramid, shown above, is especially good for the person who is constitutionally slender. Notice that fats and sweets, at the top of the pyramid, form a tiny part of the daily diet, while grains, at the base of the pyramid, form the largest part of the day's intake.

It is my observation, not necessarily scientifically based, that those of us who tend to roundness do not do well with so much grain. There are reverberations of giving grain to animals to fatten them up. For us, I recommend a low glycemic index diet:

- 2–3 protein servings daily, each coupled with a serving of a 15 percent or 20 percent fruit or vegetable (see lists, below), or 2–3 protein servings with 1 grain serving
- 1–2 tbsp. fat from vegetable sources
- 5–11 servings of 3 percent and 6 percent fruits and vegetables (see below)
- lots of water
- occasional indulgences

### *Table of Serving Sizes*

| GRAINS | PROTEINS |
|---|---|
| Bread: 1½ slices whole grain<br>1 slice white | Lean meat: 2 oz. |
| | Poultry: 2 oz. |
| Pasta: 1 c. whole grain (cooked)<br>½ c. white (cooked) | Fish: 3 oz. |
| | Whole eggs: 2 |
| Tortilla: 1 | Egg whites: 4 |
| Bagels: ½ | Low-fat cottage cheese: ½ c. |
| Rice: ½ to ¾ c. (cooked) | Low-fat yogurt: 1 c. |
| Millet: ½ to ¾ c. (cooked) | Legumes: 6 oz. |
| | Soy powder: 1 oz. |

| 15%<br>VEGETABLES | 15%<br>FRUITS | 20%<br>VEGETABLES | 20%<br>FRUITS |
|---|---|---|---|
| Artichoke: 1 | Apple: 1 med. | Beans, cooked,<br>½ c. dried | Bananas: 1 |
| Carrot: 1 raw<br>½ c. cooked | Blueberry: ½ c. | Corn: 1 cob<br>½ c. cooked | Figs: 3 fresh |
| | Cherry: ½ c. | | Prunes: 4 dried |

| 15% VEGETABLES | 15% FRUITS | 20% VEGETABLES | 20% FRUITS |
|---|---|---|---|
| Parsnip: ½ c. | Grapes: 10 | Potato (white): | Dried fruits: |
| Peas: ½ c. | Kumquats: 10 | 1 med. | 1½ oz. |
| Squash: ½ c. | Loganberry: | Potato (sweet): | |
| | ½ c. | 1 med. | |
| | Mango: 1 med. | Yams: 1 med. | |
| | Mulberry: ½ c. | | |
| | Pear: 1 med. | | |
| | Pineapple: ½ c. | | |
| | Pomegranate: | | |
| | 1 med. | | |

| 3% VEGETABLES* | 3% FRUITS* | 6% VEGETABLES* | 6% FRUITS* |
|---|---|---|---|
| Asparagus | Cantaloupe | String beans | Apricot |
| Bean sprouts | Melons | Beets | Blackberry |
| Beet greens | Rhubarb | Brussels sprouts | Black raspberry |
| Broccoli | Strawberry | Chives | Cranberry |
| Cabbage | Tomato | Collards | Grapefruit |
| Cauliflower | | Dandelion greens | Guava |
| Celery | | Eggplant | Kiwi |
| Chard | | Kale | Lemon |
| Cucumber | | Kohlrabi | Lime |
| Endive | | Leeks | Orange |
| Lettuces | | Okra | Papaya |
| Mustard | | Onion | Peach |
| greens | | Parsley | Plum |
| Radish | | Peppers | Raspberry |
| Spinach | | Pumpkin | Tangerine |
| Watercress | | Rutabaga | Ugly Fruit |
| | | Turnip | |

*Note: Serving sizes of these fruits and vegetables are limited only by personal preference; eat as much of them as you want.

# Patient's Record of Symptoms, Diagnostic Tests, and Therapies

I. SYMPTOMS (RECORD SYMPTOMS, DATES, AND SEVERITY)

Aches and pains

_____

_____

_____

_____

Breast tenderness

_____

_____

_____

_____

Dryness

_____

_____

_____

_____

Emotional turmoil

_____

_____

_____

_____

Fatigue

_____

_____

_____

_____

Fluid retention

_____

_____

_____

_____

Formication

_____

_____

_____

_____

Hot flashes, night sweats, and insomnia

_____

_____

_____

_____

Decreased libido

_____

_____

_____

_____

Menses

_____

_____

_____

_____

Migraine

_____

_____

_____

_____

Short-term memory

_____

_____

_____

_____

Urinary symptoms

_____

_____

_____

_____

_____

Vaginal symptoms

_____

_____

_____

_____


## II. DIAGNOSTIC TESTS (RECORD DATE, PLACE, AND RESULTS FOR EACH TEST)

Bone density

_____

_____

Lipids

_____

_____

Mammogram

_____

_____

Ntx

_____

_____

Occult blood

_____

_____

Pap smear

_____

_____

TSH

_____

_____

III. THERAPIES (RECORD SYMPTOMS BEING ADDRESSED AND DATE
THERAPY WAS BEGUN, ALONG WITH DOSING AND FREQUENCY;
INCLUDE RESULTS AND SIDE-EFFECTS, NOTING ADJUSTMENTS OR
DISCONTINUATION OF THERAPY)

Allopathic (Medical)

_____

_____

_____

_____

_____

Complementary

_____

_____

_____

_____

Herbal

_____

_____

_____

_____

_____

Homeopathic

---

---

---

---

---

# Resources

## Printed Materials

### BOOKLETS

"Menopause and Osteoporosis," National Osteoporosis Foundation, 1150 17th St. NW, Suite 500, Washington, DC 20036-4603
"Building Better Bones: A Guide to Active Living," The Osteoporosis Society of Canada, P.O. Box 280, Station Q, Toronto, Ontario M4T2M1 Canada

### NEWSLETTERS

*A Friend Indeed,* P.O. Box 1710, Champlain, NY 12919-1710; or, in Canada, Box 515, Place du Parc Station, Montreal, Quebec HZW 2PL Canada. Annual subscription is $30.
*Menopause News,* 2074 Union St., San Francisco, CA 94123. Annual subscription is $24.
*MenoTimes,* 1108 Irwin St., San Rafael, CA 94901. Annual subscription is $30.
*Midlife Woman,* 5129 Logan Ave. S., Minneapolis, MN 55419-1019. Annual subscription is $30.

*Additional printed materials are listed in the References at the end of this book.*

## Internet Resources

My web site is located at ⟨http://www.askyourfamilydoc.com⟩. I provide an on-line newsletter, which is updated monthly. The site and the on-line newsletter are free.

The North American Menopause Society has a site at ⟨http://www.menopause.org⟩.
Menopause Online, at ⟨http://www.menopause-online.com⟩, provides links to other useful menopause and health sites.

## Hotline

The Menopause Hotline is 1-900-370-NAMS. You will be charged $1.95 per minute for calls.

## Compounding Pharmacists and Pharmacies

### UNITED STATES

*Arizona*

Evelyn Timmons, Arizona Apothecaries, Ltd., Paradise Valley, 602-948-7065
Peter Rizzo, Prescription Lab Pharmacy, Tucson, 520-886-1035

*California*

Bob Siewert, Sierra Compounding, Auburn, 916-268-8431
Bill Altmiller, Your Drug Store, Inc., Bakersfield, 805-837-0453
Irving Reitzenstein, Valley Drug, N. Hollywood, 818-762-0686
Noel Carrico, Community Pharmacy, Sacramento, 619-355-2863
Robert Horwitz, Doc's Pharmacy & Home Health, Walnut Creek, 510-939-6312

*Colorado*

Joe Wise, Wise Pharmacy, Littleton, 303-933-8181

*Florida*

Bob Hoye, Pharmaceutical Specialties, Tampa, 813-839-8861

*Illinois*

Thomas Marks, Martin Avenue Pharmacy, Naperville,
630-355-6400

*Maryland*

Sam Giorgiou, Professional Arts Pharmacy, Baltimore,
410-747-6870

*Mississippi*

Mike Collins, Healthway Pharmacy, St. Charles, 517-865-9972

*Minnesota*

Neil Thompson, Medicine Shoppe, Minneapolis, 612-721-1623

*New Hampshire*

Ronald Petrin, Bedford Pharmacy, Bedford, 603-472-3919
George Roentsch, The Apothecary, Keene, 800-626-4379
Ron Coll, Coll's Pharmacy, Manchester, 603-623-5511
Bob Lolley, Medicine World, Nashua, 603-881-9500
Gerald Letendre, Windham Professional Pharmacy, Windham,
888-710-9525

*Texas*

Don Bottoni, Peoples Pharmacy, Austin, 512-338-5054
Phillip Pylant, Village Pharmacy, Houston, 713-464-5069

*Virginia*

Bruce Roberts, Leesburg Pharmacy, Leesburg, 703-777-5333
Andy Johnson, Biereris Pharmacy, Lexington, 540-463-2213

*Washington*

George Ballasiotes, Key Pharmacy, Kent, 206-878-3900
Bruce Ruckenbrod, Union Avenue Pharmacy, Tacoma,
253-752-2590

CANADA

*Alberta*

Ellen SanAgustin, Dermatology Centre Pharmacy, Calgary,
403-299-5808

*British Columbia*

Bob Mason, Northmount Pharmacy, North Vancouver,
604-985-8241
Lyle Sunada, Pharma-Save, Vancouver, 604-576-2888

*New Brunswick*

Peter Ford, Ford's Pharmacy, Moncton, 506-853-0830

*Ontario*

Richard Stein, Medicine Shoppe, Toronto, 416-239-3566

# Glossary

*Adaptogen:* a substance that increases the body's resistance to the adverse effects of stress and helps balance bodily functions.

*Agonist:* a substance that produces the same biological effect as another; for example, some herbs can be said to be estrogen agonists.

*Androgen:* hormones commonly thought of as being male hormones. In fact, androgens are produced by both sexes: males in the testes, liver, and adrenals, and females in the ovaries, liver, and adrenals. Women produce much less of the androgen hormones than men.

*Antagonist:* a substance that competes with another substance for binding to a receptor (for example, to an estrogen receptor) and blocks the usual biologic effect. Evista is, to some degree, an estrogen antagonist.

*Antihistamine:* a substance or drug that blocks or inhibits the release of histamine, which is a body chemical involved in the allergic response and in inflammation. Benadryl is a common antihistamine.

*Anti-inflammatory:* a substance that modifies the body's response to injury of any type—chemical, physical, or thermal. It "fights" such symptoms of inflammation as redness and swelling.

*Antioxidant:* a substance that protects against the formation of free radicals, which have been implicated in the cause of many illnesses. Vitamins C and E are examples of antioxidants.

*Antispasmodic:* a substance that acts to prevent muscle spasms.

*Atrophic vaginitis:* a condition in which the vaginal walls become thin. The vagina becomes very tender, may bleed on touch, and has a yellowish discharge that may or may not have an unpleasant odor. Atrophic vaginitis is caused by insufficient estrogen effect on the tissues of the vagina. A bacterial or yeast infection may also be present when the vagina has lost some of its natural protections.

*Bioflavonoids:* a group of pigments found in foods. This group of nutrients is essential for the functions of vitamin C.

*Bioidentical:* a pharmaceutical that exactly matches the human molecule (e.g., the soy-derived hormones are bioidentical to human hormones).

*Calcitonin:* a hormone produced by the parathyroid glands which controls calcium metabolism.

*Carcinogens:* substances that have been shown to cause cancer.

*Cholesterol:* a component of animal fats produced by the liver. It is important because it is the raw material from which the sex hormones are produced, it maintains the fluidity of cell membranes, and it is important in immunity. It is also a component of both HDL and LDL.

*Dehydroepiandrosterone (DHEA):* a mildly androgenic sex hormone produced primarily by the adrenals. It is an intermediate step in the production of testosterone and progesterone in the liver.

*Demulcent:* a substance that soothes irritated mucous membranes.

*Detoxification:* a process whereby the liver changes toxic substances into substances that are no longer toxic and can safely be eliminated from the body.

*Endorphins:* substances produced in the body that fit to the body's receptors for opiates. These substances have natural pain-relieving properties and produce a feeling of well-being.

*Equilin:* a horse estrogen.

*Fibroids:* benign tumors in the wall of the uterus which cause bleeding, pain, and pressure on the bladder.

*Formication:* an itchy feeling on the skin, as though insects were crawling on it.

*HDL:* high-density lipoproteins, the "good" cholesterol. You want this to be high.

*Hormone receptor:* a chemical configuration that binds a particular hormone in the tissues, similar to the way a specific key fits a specific lock.

*Infusion:* essentially, a tea made with fresh plant parts. Because fresh plants contain more water, larger amounts of the plant are used for an infusion than for a tea. An infusion can be made cold or hot and is often made from water or milk.

*Insomnia:* the inability to get adequate and restful sleep.

*LDL:* low-density lipoprotein, the "bad" cholesterol. You want this to be low.

*Libido:* sex drive.

*Luteal phase:* the progesterone-dominated second half of the menstrual cycle, from ovulation until bleeding.

*Menopause:* technically, the cessation of menses; actually, a process that occurs gradually, over a number of years, culminating in the cessation of menses.

*Menorrhagia:* bleeding too much during the menses. This is a form of abnormal bleeding.

*Osteopenia:* loss of bone more than one standard deviation below the mean and less than 2.5 standard deviations.

*Osteoporosis:* loss of bone greater than 2.5 standard deviations below the mean. A person with this condition has an increased risk of fracture.

*Perineum:* the area between the vagina and the anus.

*Perimenopause:* a period of time five to seven years preceding menopause, when hormonal symptoms first appear.

*Phytosterols:* plant chemicals that are very similar to human hormones.

*Postmenopause:* the time following the cessation of periods and the end of hormonal imbalances.

*Prostaglandin:* a group of hormone-like substances derived from fatty acids and having a variety of biological effects.

*SERMs:* a new class of drugs that select for some estrogen-like effects and prevent others. One example is raloxifen (Evista), which preserves bone but does not increase breast cancer risk.

*Sitz bath:* literally, sitting in a basin of warm water for its soothing qualities; the basin itself.

*Stress incontinence:* loss of control of urine while coughing, sneezing, laughing, or lifting heavy objects.

*Succussion:* very vigorous shaking used in making homeopathic dilutions.

*Tea:* a liquid drink made by steeping dried herbs in hot water.

*Tincture:* an alcohol (sometimes glycerine or vinegar) extract from an herb.

*Transdermal:* applied and absorbed through the skin.

*Withdrawal bleeding:* the period-like bleeding caused by stopping progesterone.

# References

## General

Achterberg, Jeanne. *Woman as Healer.* Shambhala Harper Perennial, 1991.

Barbach, Lonnie. *The Pause: Positive Approaches to Menopause.* New York: Dutton, 1993.

Cobb, Janine O'Leary. *Understanding Menopause.* New York: Plume, 1993.

Cone, Faye Kitchener. *Making Sense of Menopause.* New York: Simon & Schuster, 1993.

Coney, Sandra. *The Menopause Industry: How the Medical Establishment Exploits Women.* Alameda, Calif.: Hunter House, 1994.

Cutler, Winifred B., and Celso-Ramon Garcia, M.D. *Menopause: A Guide for Women and the Men Who Love Them.* New York: W. W. Norton, 1993.

Estes, Clarissa Pinkola. *Women Who Run with the Wolves.* New York: Ballantine, 1994.

Ford, Gillian. *Listening to Your Hormones.* Rocklin, Calif.: Prima Publishing, 1997.

Greenwood, Sadja, M.D. *Menopause Naturally: Preparing for the Second Half of Life.* Volcano, Calif.: Volcano Press, 1996.

Henckel, Gretchen. *The Menopause Sourcebook.* Los Angeles: Lowell House, 1994.

Jacobowitz, Ruth S. *150 Most-Asked Questions about Menopause: What Women Really Want to Know.* New York: Morrow, 1996.

Landau, Carol; Michele G. Cyr, M.D.; and Anne W. Moulton, M.D.

*The Complete Book of Menopause: Every Woman's Guide to Good Health.* New York: Perigee & Berkley, 1995.

Love, Susan, M.D. *Dr. Love's Hormone Book.* New York: Random House, 1997.

Minkin, MaryJane, M.D., and Carol V. Wright. *What Every Woman Needs to Know about Menopause: The Years Before, During, and After.* New Haven, Conn.: Yale University Press, 1996.

Nachtigall, Lila E., M.D.; Robert D. Nachtigall, M.D.; and Joan Rattner Heilman. *What Every Woman Should Know: Staying Healthy after Forty.* New York: Warner Books, 1996.

Nachtigall, Lila E., M.D., and Joan Rattner Heilman. *Estrogen: The Facts Can Save Your Life.* New York: Harper, 1995.

Notelovitz, Morris, M.D., and Diana Tonnessen. *Menopause and Midlife Health.* New York: St. Martin's Press, 1993.

Ojeda, Linda. *Menopause without Medicine.* Alameda, Calif.: Hunter House, 1995.

Sand, Gayle. *Is It Hot in Here or Is It Me?* New York: Harper, 1994.

Schiff, Isaac, M.D., and Ann B. Parson. *Menopause.* New York: Times Books, 1996.

Sheehy, Gail. *The Silent Passage.* New York: Random House, 1998.

Rako, Susan, M.D. *The Hormone of Desire.* New York: Harmony Books, 1996.

Taylor, Dena, and Amber Sumrall. *Women of the Fourteenth Moon.* Freedom, Calif.: Crossing, 1991.

Teaff, Nancy Lee, M.D., and Kim Wright Wiley. *Perimenopause— Preparing for the Change: Guide to the Early Stages of Menopause and Beyond.* Rocklin, Calif.: Prima Publishing, 1996.

Utian, Wulf, M.D. *Managing Your Menopause.* New York: Prentice Hall, 1990.

Vliet, Judith, M.D. *Screaming to Be Heard.* New York: Evans, 1995.

Walker, Barbara G. *The Crone: Women of Age, Wisdom, and Power.* New York: Harper, 1998.

Weed, Sussun S. *Menopausal Years: The Wise Woman Way.* Woodstock, N.Y.: Ashtree Publishing, 1992.

West, Stanley, M.D., and Paula Dranov. *The Hysterectomy Hoax.* New York: Doubleday, 1994.

# Herbal

Brinker, Francis J., N.D. *Toxicology of Botanical Medicine.* Sandy, Ore.: Eclectic Medical Publishing, 1989.
Brown, Donald J., and Eric Yarnell, N.D. *Phytotherapy Research Compendium.* Seattle: Natural Product Research Consultants, 1997.
Hoffman, David. *Holistic Herbal.* Rockport, Mass.: Element, 1996.
Kloss, Jethro. *Back to Eden.* Place: Woodbridge Press, 1981.
Lust, John, N.D. *The Herb Book.* New York: Bantam, 1974.
Murrary, Michael T., N.D. *The Healing Power of Herbs.* Rocklin, Calif.: Prima Publishing, 1995.
Tyler, Varro E. *The Honest Herbal.* New York: Pharmaceutical Products Press, 1993.
Weed, Sussun S. *Menopausal Years: The Wise Woman Way.* Woodstock, N.Y.: Ashtree Publishing, 1992.
Weiss, Rudolf R., M.D. *Herbal Medicine.* Sandy, Ore.: Eclectic Medical Publishing, 1988.

# Homeopathic

Bach, Edward, M.D., and F. J. Wheeler, M.D. *The Bach Flower Remedies.* New Canaan, Conn.: Keats Publishing, 1979.
Boger, C. M. *A Synoptic Key of the Materia Medica.* New Delhi: B. Jain Publishing, 1984.
Kent, J. T., M.D. *Lectures on Homeopathic Materia Medica.* New Delhi: Homeopathic Publications, 1911.
Kent, J. T., M.D. *Repertory of the Homeopathic Materia Medica.* New Delhi: World Homeopathic Links, 1983.
Lessell, Colin B. *Homeopathy for Physicians.* Wellingborough, Northamptonshire: Thorsons Publishers, 1983.

Smith, Trevor, M.D. *Homeopathic Medicine*. New York: Thorson Publishing, 1983.

Weiner, B., and Goss, K. *The Complete Book of Homeopathy*. New York: Bantam, 1982.

## Estriol

Ahlstrom K., et al. "Effect of combined treatment with phenylpropanolamine and estriol, compared with estriol treatment alone, in postmenopausal women with stress urinary incontinence." *Gynecologic and Obstetric Investigation* 30 (1990): 37–43.

Akkad, A., et al. "Carotid plaque regression on oestrogen replacement: a pilot study." *European Journal of Vascular and Endovascular Surgery* 11 (1996): 347–48.

Arnold, W. P.; B. J. Pennings; and P. C. van de Kerkhof. "The induction of epidermal ornithine decarboxylase following UV-B irradiation is inhibited by estriol." *Acta Dermato-Venereologica* 73 (1993): 92–93.

Canez, M. S.; K. H. Lee; and D. L. Olive. "Progesterone and estrogens." *Infertility and Reproductive Medical Clinics of North America* 3 (1992): 59–78.

Doren, M., et al. "Superior compliance and efficacy of continuous combined oral estrogen-progesterone replacement therapy in postmenopausal women." *American Journal of Obstetrics and Gynecology* 173 (1995): 1446–51.

Follingstad, A. H. "Estriol: the forgotten estrogen?" *Journal of the American Medical Association* 239 (1978): 29–30.

Haines, C., et al. "Effect of oral estradiol on Lp(a) and other lipoproteins in postmenopausal women. A randomized, double-blind, placebo-controlled, crossover study." *Archives of Internal Medicine* 156 (1996): 866–72.

Hawthorn, R. J., et al. "The endometrial status of women on long-term continuous combined hormone replacement therapy." *British Journal of Obstetrics and Gynaecology* 98 (1991): 939–40.

Heithecker, R., et al. "Plasma estriol levels after intramuscular injections of estriol and two of its esters." *Hormone Research* 35 (1991): 234–38.

Henriksson, L., et al. "A comparative multicenter study of the effects of continuous low-dose estradiol released from a new vaginal ring versus estradiol vaginal pessaries in postmenopausal women with symptoms and signs of urogenital atrophy." *American Journal of Obstetrics and Gynecology* 171 (1994): 624–32.

Holland, E. F.; A. T. Leather; and J. W. Studd. "Increase in bone mass of older postmenopausal women with low bone mineral density after one year of percutaneous estradiol implants." *British Journal of Obstetrics and Gynaecology* 102 (1995): 238–42.

Iida, K.; A. Imai; and T. Tamaya. "Estriol binding in uterine corpus cancer and in normal uterine tissues." *General Pharmacology* 22 (1991): 491–93.

Iosif, C. S. "Effects of prolonged administration of estriol on the lower genito-urinary tract in postmenopausal women." *Archives of Gynecology and Obstetrics* 251 (1992): 115–20.

Kainz, C., et al. "When applied to facial skin, does estrogen ointment have systemic effects?" *Archives of Gynecology and Obstetrics* 253 (1993): 71–74.

Lauritzen, C. "The female climacteric syndrome: significance, problems, and treatment." *Acta Obstetrica et Gynaecologica Scandinavia* 51 (1976): 49–61.

Lauritzen, C. "The management of the pre-menopausal and the post-menopausal patient." *Front. Hormone Research* 22 (1973): 21.

Lemon, H. M. "Estriol prevention of mammary carcinoma induced by 12-dimethyl-benzanthracen and procarbazine." *Cancer Research* 35 (1975): 1311–53.

Lemon, H. M., et al. "Inhibition of radiogenic mammary carcinoma in rats by estriol or tamoxifen." *Cancer* 63 (1989): 1685–92.

Levitz, M., et al. "Relationship between the concentration of estriol sulfate and estrone sulfate in human breast cyst fluid." *Journal of Clinical Endocrinology and Metabolism* 75 (1992): 726–29.

Molander, U., et al. "A health care program for the investigation and treatment of elderly women and urinary incontinence and related urogenital symptoms." *Acta Obstetrica et Gynaecologica Scandinavia* 70 (1991): 137–42.

Myrup, B.; G. F. Jensen; and P. McNair. "Cardiovascular risk factors during estrogen-norethindrone and cholecalciferol treatment." *Archives of Internal Medicine* 152 (1992): 2265–68.

Othman, Y. S., and R. E. Oakey. "Why so much estriol? A comparison of the aromatization of androstenedione and 16-alpha-hydroxyandrostenedione when incubated alone or together with human placental microsomes." *Journal of Endocrinology* 148 (1996): 399–407.

Pasqualini, J. R.; C. Gelly; and B. L. Nguyen. "Metabolism and biologic response of estrogen sulfates in hormone-dependent and hormone-independent mammary cancer cell lines. Effect of antiestrogens." *Annals of the New York Academy of Sciences* 595 (1990): 106–16.

Raz, R., and W. E. Stamm. "A controlled trial of intravaginal estriol in postmenopausal women with recurrant urinary tract infections. *New England Journal of Medicine* 329 (1993): 753–56.

Ritter, J. K.; Y. Y. Sheen; and I. S. Owens. "Cloning and expression of human liver UDP-glucuronosyltransferase in COS-1 cells. 3,4-catechol estrogens and estriol as primary substrates." *Journal of Biological Chemistry* 265 (1990): 7900–7906.

Saure, A. "Randomized comparison of a new estradiol-releasing vaginal ring versus estriol vaginal pessaries (letter). *American Journal of Obstetrics and Gynecology* 173 (1995): 670–71.

Seshadri, R., et al. "Conversion to estriol in 'normal,' benign, and malignant human breast tissues." *Journal of Cancer Research and Clinical Oncology* 116 (1990): 271–74.

Tadmor, O. P., et al. "The effects of two fixed hormonal replacement therapy protocols on blood lipid profiles." *European Journal of Obstetrics, Gynaecology, and Reproductive Biology* 46 (1992): 109–16.

Tepper, R., et al. "Estrogen replacement in postmenopausal women: are we currently overdosing our patients?" *Gynecologic and Obstetric Investigation* 38 (1994): 113–16.

Tonstad, S. "Combined hormone replacement therapy with oestradiol and nor-ethsterone acetate: effects on hyperlipidaemia." *British Journal of Obstetrics and Gynaecology* 103, suppl. (May 1996): 45–48.

Ulrich, L. G. "Accumulated knowledge of Kliogest safety aspects." *British Journal of Obstetrics and Gynaecology* 13 (1996): 99–102; 102–3.

van der Linden, M. C., et al. "The effect of estriol on the cytology of urethra and vagina in post-menopausal women with genitourinary symptoms." *European Journal of Obstetrics, Gynaecology, and Reproductive Biology* 51 (1993): 29–33.

Vooijs, G. P., and T. B. Geurts. "Review of the endometrial safety during intravaginal treatment with estriol." *European Journal of Obstetrics, Gynaecology, and Reproductive Biology* 62 (1995): 101–6.

Weiderpass, E.; J. A. Baron; H. O. Adami; C. Magnusson; A. Lindgren; R. Bergstrom; N. Correia; and I. Persson. "Low-potency oestrogen and risk of endometrial cancer: a case-control study." *Lancet* 353 (1999): 1824–28.

Writing Group for the PEPI Trial. "Effects of estrogen or estrogen/progestin regimens on heart disease risk factors in postmenopausal women." *Journal of the American Medical Association* 273 (1995): 199–208.

Yang, T. S., et al. "Efficacy and safety of estriol replacement therapy for climacteric women." *American Journal of Obstetrics and Gynecology* 173 (1995): 670–71.

## Hormone Replacement Therapy

Andrews, W. C. "Menopause." *Menopause: The Journal of the North American Menopause Society* 2 (1994): 59–65.

Avis, N. E., and C. Johannes. "Socioeconomic status and HRT use."

*Menopause: The Journal of the North American Menopause Society* 5 (1998): 137–39.

Barrett-O'Connor, E., and D. Goodman-Gruen. "Prospective study of endogenous sex hormones and fatal cardiovascular disease in postmenopausal women." *British Medical Journal* 311 (1995): 1193–96.

Bartman, B. A., and E. Moy. "Racial differences in estrogen use among middle-aged and older women." *Women's Health Issues* 8 (1998): 32–44.

Beral., V. E. Banks; and G. Reeves. "Evidence from randomized trials on the long-term effects of hormone replacement therapy." *Lancet* 360 (2002): 942–44.

Berman, R. S., et al. "Compliance of women in taking estrogen replacement therapy." *Journal of Women's Health* 5 (1996): 213–20.

Cagnacci, A., et al. "Depression and anxiety in climacteric women: role of hormone replacement therapy." *Menopause: The Journal of the North American Menopause Society* 4 (1997): 206–12.

Canez, M. S.; K. H. Lee; and D. L. Olive. "Progesterones and estrogens." *Infertility and Reproduction Medical Clinics of North America* 3 (1992): 59–78.

Cauley, J. A., et al. "Estrogen replacement therapy and mortality among older women." *Archives of Internal Medicine* 157 (1997): 2181–87.

Chakmakjian, A. H., and N. Y. Zachariah. "Bioavailability of progesterone with different modes of administration." *Journal of Reproductive Medicine* 32 (1987): 443–47.

Chlebowski, R. T., et al., for the WHI Investigators. "Influence of estrogen plus progestin on breast cancer and mammography in healthy postmenopausal women: the Women's Health Initiative randomized trial." *Journal of the American Medical Association* 289 (2003): 3243–53.

Cobleigh, M. A., et al. "Estrogen replacement therapy in breast cancer survivors." *Journal of the American Medical Association* 272 (1994): 540–45.

Colditz, G. A., et al. "Type of postmenopausal hormone use and risk of breast cancer: 12-year follow-up from the Nurses' Health Study." *Cancer Causes and Control* 3 (1992): 433–39.

Colditz, G. A., et al. "The use of estrogens and progestins and the risk of breast cancer in postmenopausal women." *New England Journal of Medicine* 332 (1995): 1589–93.

Da Souza, M. J., et al. "A comparison of the effect of synthetic and micronized hormone replacement therapy on bone mineral density and biochemical markers of bone metabolism." *Menopause: The Journal of the North American Menopause Society* 3 (1996): 140–48.

de Lignieres, B.; L. Dennerstein; and T. Backstrom. "Influence of route of administration on progesterone metabolism." *Maturitas* 21 (1995): 251–57.

DiSaia, P. J., et al. "Hormone replacement therapy in breast cancer survivors: a cohort study." *American Journal of Obstetrics and Gynecology* 174 (1996): 1494–98.

Dupont, A., et al. "Comparative endocrinological and clinical effects of percutaneous estradiol and oral conjugated estrogens as replacement therapy in menopausal women." *Maturitas* 13 (1991): 297–311.

Eden, J. A. "A case-control study of combined continuous estrogen-progestin replacement therapy among women with a personal history of breast cancer." *Menopause: The Journal of the North American Menopause Society* 2 (1995): 67–72.

Ettinger, B.; A. Pressman; and C. Bradley. "Comparison of continuation of postmenopausal hormone replacement therapy: transdermal vs. oral estrogen." *Menopause: The Journal of the North American Menopause Society* 5 (1998): 152–57.

Ettinger, B., et al. "Reducing mortality associated with long-term postmenopausal estrogen therapy." *Obstetrics and Gynecology* 87 (1996): 6–12.

Gillet, J. Y., et al. "Induction of amenorrhoea during hormone replacement therapy: optimal micronized progesterone dose. A multicenter study." *Maturitas* 19 (1994): 103–15.

Grady, D., et al. "Hormone therapy to prevent disease and prolong life in postmenopausal women." *Annals of Internal Medicine* 117 (1992): 1010–16.

Grodstein, F., et al. "Postmenopausal hormone therapy and mortality." *New England Journal of Medicine* 336 (1997): 1769–75.

Hargrove, J. T., et al. "Menopausal hormone replacement therapy with continuous daily oral micronized estradiol and progesterone." *Obstetrics and Gynecology* 73 (1989): 606–12.

Hargrove, J. T., and K. G. Oseen. "An alternative method of hormone replacement therapy using the natural sex steroids." *Menopause: The Journal of the North American Menopause Society* 6 (1995): 653–74.

Hawthorn, R. J. S.; K. Spowart; and D. M. Hart. "The endometrial status of women on long-term continuous combined hormone replacement therapy." *British Journal of Obstetrics and Gynaecology* 98 (1991): 939–42.

Henriksson, L., et al. "A comparative study of the effects of continuous low-dose estradiol released from a new vaginal ring versus estriol vaginal pessaries in postmenopausal women with symptoms and signs of urogenital atophy." *American Journal of Obstetrics and Gynecology* 171 (3): 624–32.

Hirvonen, E., et al. "Effects of transdermal oestrogen therapy in postmenopausal women: a comparative study of an oestradiol gel and an oestradiol delivering patch." *British Journal of Obstetrics and Gynaecology* 16 (1997): 26–31.

Hirvonen, E., et al. "Transdermal oestradiol gel in the treatment of the climacterium: a comparison with oral therapy." *British Journal of Obstetrics and Gynaecology* 16 (1997): 19–25.

McManus, J., et al. "The effect of various oestrogens and progestogens on the susceptibility of low density lipoproteins to oxidation in vitro." *Maturitas* 25 (1996): 125–31.

Metka, M., et al. "The role of prolactin in the menopause." *Maturitas* 20 (1995): 151–54.

Million Women Study Collaborators. "Breast cancer and hormone-replacement therapy in the Million Women Study." *Lancet* 362 (2003): 419–27.

Montgomery, J. C., et al. "Effect of Oestrogen and testosterone implants on psychological disorders in the climacteric." *Lancet* 7 Feb. (1987): 297–99.

Moyer, D. L., et al. "Prevention of endometrial hyperplasia by progesterone during long-term estradiol replacement: influence of bleeding pattern and secretory changes." *Fertility and Sterility* 59 (1993): 992–97.

Prestwood, K. M., et al. "Ultralow-dose micronized 17-β-estradiol and bone density and bone metabolism in older women: a randomized controlled trial." *Journal of the American Medical Association* 290 (2003): 1042–48.

Scarabin, P.-Y., et. al. "Differential association of oral and transdermal oestrogen replacement therapy with venous thromboembolism risk." *Lancet* 363 (2003): 428–32.

Shen, L., et al. "Alkylation of 2-deoxynucleosides and DNA by the premarin metabolite 4-hydroxyequilenin semiquinone radical." *Chemical Research in Toxicology*, website release, Jan. 23, 1998.

Stampfer, M. J., and F. Grodstein. "Colorectal cancer: does postmenopausal estrogen use reduce the risk?" *Menopause Management* 8 (1999): 8–11.

Studd, J., et al. "Efficacy and acceptability of Intranasal 17-β-oestradiol for menopausal symptoms." *Lancet* 8 May (1999); 353(9164): 1574–78.

Tadmor, O. P., et al. "The effects of two fixed hormonal replacement therapy protocols on blood lipid profiles." *European Journal of Obstetrics, Gynaecology, and Reproductive Biology* 46 (1992): 109–16.

Tepper, R., et al. "Estrogen replacement in postmenopausal women: are we currently overdosing our patients?" *Gynecologic and Obstetric Investigation* 38 (1994): 113–16.

Utian, W. H. "HRT and the HERS Findings—has the ground shifted?" *Menopause Management* 7 (1998): 5.

Weiderpass, E., et al. "Low-potency oestrogen and risk of endometrial cancer." *Lancet* 29 May (1999); 353(9167): 1824–28.

Wren, B. G.; L. B. Brown; and D. A. Routledge. "Differential clinical response to oestrogens after menopause." *Medical Journal of Australia* 2 (1982): 305–52.

Writing Group for the PEPI Trial. "Effects of estrogen or estrogen/ progestin regimens on heart disease risk factors in postmenopausal women." *Journal of the American Medical Association* 273 (1995): 199–208.

Writing Group for the PEPI Trial. "Effects of hormone replacement therapy on endometrial histology in postmenopausal women." *Journal of the American Medical Association* 275 (1996): 370–75.

Writing Group for the Women's Health Initiative Investigators. "Risks and benefits of estrogen plus progestin in healthy postmenopausal women: principal results from the Women's Health Initiative randomized controlled trial." *Journal of the American Medical Association* 288 (2002): 321–33.

# Index